Robert Netherway

OUT OF THE
DARK

Making the best of a
life with limited vision

MEREO

Mereo Books

2nd Floor, 6-8 Dyer Street, Cirencester, Gloucestershire, GL7 2PF
An imprint of Memoirs Books. www.mereobooks.com
and www.memoirsbooks.co.uk

Out of the Dark

978-1-86151-980-1

First published in Great Britain in 2021
by Mereo Books, an imprint of Memoirs Books.

Copyright ©2021

The address for Memoirs Books can be
found at www.mereobooks.com

Mereo Books Ltd. Reg. No. 12157152

Typeset in 11/15pt Century Schoolbook
by Wiltshire Associates.
Printed and bound in Great Britain

Acknowledgements

In writing this book I would like to thank all those people who contributed ideas and encouraged me to continue writing when the going got tough.

I would particularly like to thank my friend Vicky who edited it so diligently, also my family and other friends who were curious enough to read it.

Bob Netherway
March 2021

Preface

This book is the story of a boy who was born blind. Robert Netherway was born in 1948 and brought up on a farm in rural Devonshire, a few miles west of the city of Exeter. After pioneering eye surgery on the new NHS he gained sufficient sight to work on his father's hill farm. He attended a school for visually impaired children and embarked on training for a career.

There is also a look at the author's philosophy as he learned to cope with adulthood, and how he overcame the challenge of coming to come to terms with losing his sight again permanently in later life.

Contents

1   Early Years 1

2   Life on the farm 10

3   Village life 38

4   Learning challenges 48

5   The Swinging Sixties 59

6   College days 66

7   Training for a career 92

8   Personal issues 98

9   Riding the air waves 106

10 A home of my own 114

11 Making music 120

12 A new millennium 132

13 Closing thoughts 141

CHAPTER 1

Early years

❖

My father

My father, Robert Vaughn Netherway, was born on 3rd September 1915, to Thomas and Emily Netherway. There were three children, my father Robert, Bernard and Edith. Their home was at Lime Tree Road, Plymouth. When dad was only a little boy he told me that he would go out in the mornings to get the cows in for milking.

In about 1930, when the family were older, Grandpa moved the family to Dawlish, where he had a butchery business which was the foundation for Farm Barton where we lived later. The two boys had different ideas of the work they wanted to do when they were older. Dad had very fixed ideas about what he wanted to do, but Bernard was not keen on farming, and wanted to be a civil engineer. This difference of opinion caused friction between them.

Grandpa bought the farm in the middle of the recession of 1931, a shrewd decision for his business.

Edith met Lennard, who like her was interested in amateur opera and other stage productions, and that led to their connection with the Theatre Royal in in Exeter. During the Second World War, Dad was in a reserved occupation, so he stayed on the farm, serving in the Home Guard at night. He told me that being on duty on Exminster Marshes could be very hard in winter.

In 1940 he met my mother, who had left London for a more peaceful life, and they met the day after she had moved to Exeter. They married in December 1941.

Bernard did a lot of work on the farm plus improving the house at Farm Barton and another at Pitt Farm, adjoining Barton. We children were born during the late 1940s, and we had a good family upbringing despite all the shortages that followed the war.

Dad pursued his passion for singing in the voluntary choir in Exeter Cathedral into the 60s and appeared on 'Songs of Praise' one Christmas.

When Grandpa died my father took over, but he was not able to modernise the business and the farm stayed a small enterprise.

Dad died on August 26th 2008, at just after 6.30 in the evening.

Mum

My mother was born on the 11th April 1915. She stood approximately 5ft 6in tall and was stockily built. Dad, who stood about 5ft 9 ins tall, was slim and very fit, as he did manual work all his life.

Mum's first job had been with a firm of solicitors in London, where she grew up. Dad was born in Plymouth and lived there until he was 15, when his parents moved to Dawlish for the family butchery business. Mum soon decided that she wanted to go into nursing and became qualified in radiology –

X-rays. She continued to work in that field until she met Dad in 1940. They were married in December 1941, and the first of four children, three girls and a boy, myself. Ruth was born in the terrible winter of 1947, on 16th February. My two younger sisters were Christine, born August 30th 1950, and Mary, who arrived on October 12th 1956. I was born on May 18th 1948.

During the Second World War the bombing got so bad that Mum decided to leave London and find another job in a smaller town. An advertisement had been placed in a national newspaper for nursing staff to go and work in Devon, and she decided to take up a post at Exeter's Royal Devon and Exeter General Hospital. There she met another nurse and shared a room in the nurses' home. Her friend knew Dad but did not want to go out with him and suggested that Mum might like to go instead, which she did. They had some dates together and got married the following December, 1941.

Life on a farm just outside a provincial city was a world away from life in Ilford in Greater London. It lacked sophistication and was basic, but it afforded safety as the village was three miles away from the city of Exeter, which did suffer some very destructive air raids.

When the war was over Mum very soon started a family, as described earlier. Work on the farm was part of her life. She not only did all the housework but contributed a lot to the work on the farm, being involved with the lambing during the winter and haymaking in summer.

Mum had traded a professional life for rural farm life. She always said that she would never go back to London, and she never did so except when her father died in the late 60s, then her mother later. Both her parents made visits to see her in Devon of course and at one time they moved to Exmouth, but they did not stay for very long before returning to London. My mother was 74 when she died.

Life together

My mother and father shared an interest in music. Dad had been attending the voluntary choir in Exeter Cathedral for a long time, maybe since before the war. Mum had an interest in singing from the time she had been at school.

Dad kept extremely fit doing manual work on the farm. He had a somewhat dry sense of humour. Most of the time his dress was that of a typical farmer: flat cap, overalls and on cold nights an army greatcoat. But on Sundays and for choir he dressed very smartly and wore a trilby hat.

Mum, who was always working outside as well as in, did dress for the occasion. I don't remember for instance her having a hairdo except for when the girls got married. Her usual style was to wear her hair in a bun at the back, and that hardly ever changed.

Mum did not have a sense of humour to speak of. Her outlook on life was rather sad and she tended to look on the negative side. Her work outside was to keep the flower garden, as well as the vegetable garden. In the summer she would help with the hay, and she always supplied us with a lovely tea out in the hay field.

My life was destined to be very different from those of my siblings. To begin with an infection in the womb caused by the rubella virus was to have a profound influence on my early development and as a consequence, my schooling. Fortunately my parents were sensible and took advice as to what would be best for me.

When Ruth was older she developed a strong interest in botany and related subjects. After leaving secondary school she went to Roll College in Exmouth, then went to a course in Dartington Hall in South Devon under the tuition of Terry Underhill, who led the gardening operation at the college.

My next sister, Christine, was born on 30th August 1950 and went to Ide Primary School in the village of Ide near Exeter. She later went on to study art at Exeter Art College.

Mary was last to be born, on 12th October 1956. After school she went on to a career in nursing at Bristol Royal infirmary.

My first visit to a hospital took place was when I was only five months old. My condition, congenital rubella, meant that I was born blind due to an opaque film over my eyes. My first memories were of not being able to see at all, but the operations that were performed within the new NHS by Mr Rutter enabled me to see some very vague images. I remember being laid on the kitchen table and seeing the gas light above my head and hearing the hiss of the gas as it burned. I am eternally grateful to Mr Rutter for performing the necessary procedure in order that I might see.

Over many years he carried out more operations on my tiny eyes until when I was 15-16 years of age, and with the right glasses, I was able to see very well. There is an irony in that if my parents could have waited until I had been about 10 years old, Mr Rutter could have performed what is called a 'senile cataract operation', in which the opaque substance, which hardens, could have been removed without damaging the lenses of my eyes, giving me much better sight. But my parents' anxiety is understandable and I can appreciate why they wanted to get the operation done as soon as possible, as without it I would not have learned some of the essential knowledge we acquire during the early years. If I had been sent to a school for the totally blind I would have developed a very different mindset from the one I have now.

Pairs of glasses came and went, and at first I would keep throwing them away until eventually I accepted that they were a benefit to me. Once I reached my teens I was able to read newspaper headlines and could read about four rows down the eye chart.

When I was five my mother took me to school for the first time. Back then there were no pre-school nurseries where children could meet other children for the first time, so it must have been a big shock for me to meet them, never mind the teachers.

Looking back at my start in life on a farm with all the shortages that we had to contend with at the time, I think I was lucky to be born into such a resourceful family.

CHAPTER 2

Life on the farm

◆§ ··•·· §◆

Making hay

When you are a little boy living on a farm you are expected to join in with the family activities and do your share of the work. This you can regard as fun or slave labour, according to your point of view.

One job I hated was cleaning the milking machine and another was mucking out the cows after milking. The smell gave me quite bad nausea, particularly after I had just had tea. On the other hand there were some jobs I loved. Once the hay had been mown it was left to dry for the day and then turned and rowed up ready for the bailer. The bailer would arrive usually later that day or maybe the following morning and the bailing would begin. On some occasions my job would be to ride on the back of the bailer, where the bales came out, to make sure that the cords were sufficiently tight. If they were not, I would shout to the driver, as quite often the knotter was at fault. Some things never change, do they!

With the bailing done the bales were stood up in small groups ready for collecting. This could be hard work on a hot day and loading a trailer of bales is a thing you have to take particular care with, as if it is not done carefully and methodically they will soon fall apart.

Having loaded the trailer we would begin the journey back to the yard. During the ride back I would be on the top of the load and would have to be careful to remember to duck when the trailer passed under overhanging branches, as I would be knocked off if I was not quick enough.

Having arrived back at home, Cousin John or whoever was driving the tractor would back the loaded trailer into the yard and park it next to the hayloft where we were going to put the hay. We had an elevator which was a big improvement on the early days when it was done manually with a two-prong pick. One or two lads would put the bales on the elevator and I would be at the top to receive them. I then passed the bales back to another of the team who would stack them neatly ready for the winter when they were needed. Under the slate roof on a hot day it was a gruelling job up there in suffocating heat.

Quite often dad would drive down to the Royal Oak and buy a crate of ale for the lads as it was such thirsty work. A perfect end to a perfect day..

The corn harvest

Just as with the hay, the corn came a month later if weather conditions were right. One of the most important requirements for harvesting corn, be it barley, wheat or oats, is the moisture content. Most small farmers like us didn't possess the measuring equipment to do this important test, so we relied on the seed mill to do this for us. We used to go to a very well-known mill in the nearby town of Crediton six miles away from Farm Barton, along the narrow lanes then down a steep hill into the town.

Once at the mill the man who carried out the test for us kept the necessary gear in the office, as the mill was so noisy we could not have heard what he said about the sample's moisture. If the value of the sample was below 10 percent the mill would take it, but if it was higher then for every percent over 10 they would impose a surcharge for drying, which is an expensive process.

In the early days, when I was old enough, I used to ride on the combine, which was one of the first self-propelled machines brought over from the USA under the lease-lend scheme after World War 2. The one sent to us was a Massey Harris 727. My job was to stand on the platform with an open sack and fill the bag up so it was nearly full, then pass it to my cousin John, who stitched the top up and then put it down the chute at the back. It was a far cry from the method of harvesting by today's monsters, which can cost upwards of £400,000!

The dangers of farms

My early years on the farm at and school were days of innocence. I was taking in so many new things in my life, some of which I still carry around in my mind and regard them as merely growing pains. Then there are memories which have caused me to appreciate the significance of the situation I was in. For instance, living on a farm I soon learned about danger as there was plenty of it. The animals could be dangerous, particularly if they had young. Cows would attack to protect their young, and if there was a bull in the field you could definitely expect trouble.

When you are three years old, full of curiosity and living on a farm wandering away from your home and not under your mum's watchful eyes can be dangerous. My first recollection is of running into a nearby lane and hitting my head on something very hard and falling backwards. What had happened was that the sun was low and I had failed to see that one of the grown-ups had put a tree trunk across the open gateway to prevent people or animals from wandering into the field.

As time went on there were more hazards, You would not think that baling hay could be dangerous, but I heard quite recently that some time in the 1980s a farmer or farm worker who had a problem with a baler forgot to turn off the PTO (power take off) on the tractor when he went round to the front of the baler to dislodge something that had got into the pickup tines of the machine. His clothes were caught by the tines and he was unceremoniously dragged into the mechanism and baled.

There are plenty of other things on the farm which can "get you." Mowing machines have a bed of triangular knives which are very close to the ground, and if the unaware are not vigilant they can have their ankles cut off. Fire is another danger. Quite often there are reports of barn or hay rick fires which a lot of people assume are caused by vandals or lit cigarette ends, but very often they are caused by spontaneous combustion, rather like when a compost heap heats up and when dry will burst into flames. Some children like to play by making a den of bales, but if they are playing with matches that is inviting disaster.

Farm machinery was something you had to learn about. You had to be sure that the operator of machines, tractors etc, was aware that you could be in its way. Then there were the natural dangers, like flood and fire. For a child these could be a real danger and quite unexpected. Until recently chemicals were another hazard on farms.

Many toxic chemicals are used on farms. Dioxin, which is used for killing weeds or anything which is not wanted in the growing of crops, can also kill humans and animals. Until the early 2000s farmers used to use Cymag to gas the massive populations of rabbits found on farms. It was banned by the Government, as it was so dangerous that the instructions on the tin said that if you had contact with this nerve agent, a physician must be summoned within three minutes. I was taught about this at an early age.

You should never go into a field containing cows if they have their young with them. They can be just as dangerous as any bull, and will protect their offspring. Cows have very poor eyesight but that does not mean they can't do a lot of damage if they think their calves are in danger.

Later in life, when I reached my late teens, I began to despair at some things that I thought ought to happen but did not, such as relationships with girls. I concluded that I was too young to get involved with these activities, and it would be better to leave them until later in life.

By the age of 13 I could drive a tractor, and by 20 I could ride a motorbike and drive our family car, an Austin A65 Farina, which was grey with a lighter grey stripe along the side. It was a cumbersome thing to drive at slow speed, a bit like a tank, and the driver's seat was at an odd angle, but at higher speeds it was not too bad.

Most of the farm was devoted to sheep, which, as an infant I did not have great interest in, but we did have some cows which did arouse my curiosity. There were only a few of them, about 10, and they had to be milked twice a day.

When I was older I would go out with my mother across the fields, and that was when I saw the sheep.

At lambing time mum used to get tame lambs which the mother had rejected, so she would have to rear them herself by feeding them on cows' milk from the bottle.

There were a few fields, such as Catherine Field and Bushes, which had a boundary with the road that led you towards Exeter, Bushes being the last one. One small field, Frenche's close below Catherine Field, was steep like all the others and ended right down the bottom of Farm Barton near the brook. One of the great assets of the farm was that it was south facing, so it got the sun from early in the morning till late evening in summer, an important consideration for growing crops, and for the wellbeing of the stock in the winter.

Nearer to the farmhouse was a small field we called the Platt. It only amounted to about one acre, and was used to graze sheep, and we had a small enclosure there for some geese. In front of the house we had a large garden which mum looked after in addition to that there was another garden to the right of the house we called the "Top Garden" which my eldest sister Ruth had grown a lot of polyanthus and other flowers. Trees there were, cypresses and another we called a deoda.

At the back of the farmhouse was one more small patch of land where I had a garden in which I had grown a few flowers and some vegetables.

Farm sales

A regular part of farm life was the farm sales. From time to time we would be notified of a sale in the area. These sales were conducted by local auctioneers on behalf of farmers who might be selling for a number of reasons such as bereavement, or more commonly, bankruptcy. Only a few sold up due to expansion.

Arriving at the farm, dad would park our olive green Morris Oxford and make our way to the farmyard and buildings, where the auctioneer might already be selling the livestock – he usually did that first so they could be moved off the farm quickly. Most of these farms were like our own, small operations with perhaps ten or twelve dairy cows and a few sheep. Not all were small – some were big concerns – but this was mid-Devon in the early 60s, and the local economy dictated that small farms prevailed. 'Come on gentlemen, what am I bid for this fine Friesian, £150? £125? Somebody start the bidding? You sir on my right, start the bidding, give me an offer.' A voice says '£100'. And so it gets going at a rapid pace if the animal looks to be worth the offer.

Livestock sold, we would all move out of the yard into the nearby field where the deadstock awaited the same treatment.

Farm machinery is sought after by farmers who may not have that particular implement of their own. Quite often you see the same piece of equipment at another sale just a few weeks later, because it failed to reach its reserve price the last time. The biggest item we bought was an IH (International Harvester) self-powered hay baler. We got several seasons out of it before the engine gave up, and no amount of repairs would keep it going. In the end I dismantled part of it and got the local scrap merchant to do the rest.

There would also be sundries such as hand tools, and a few curios (like the Field Marshall), such as a device called a 'zollop.' The zollop, the name that dad gave it, was a kidney-shaped bucket that the user held towards their waist. It would be filled with seed for hand sowing, or fertiliser. It had a handle on the front to enable the user to hold it towards themselves. No shoulder straps though. It's hard to believe that nobody in those days had sufficient imagination to put straps on the zollop, like a pair of braces, to give the worker two free hands!

There were also the other usual hand tools like giant corkscrews for boring holes in gateposts to fit the hangers. Nowadays, gateposts are made of plastic and the holes are pre-drilled, and the hand corkscrew device has been replaced by a tractor-mounted machine that drills the holes for the posts and does it very efficiently indeed.

We always felt a bit sad going to these sales as they represented the culmination of some poor farmer's efforts, often over a lifetime in difficult circumstances, such as making a living on poor soil, or the ups and downs of the market place, but they were a fact of life and unless the farmer and the farm (like ours) adapted to modern conditions they simply went out of business.

Market day

At about 9 am most Fridays, the cattle lorry would arrive and reverse down the concrete slope that was the entrance to the yard. First, the driver would undo the two locks which kept the back of the lorry securely shut, then he would proceed to lower it to the ground to form a loading ramp. Next he would open the gates which were behind the ramp and place them so that the animals did not get through the gaps either side of the lorry.

Animals have instinct; they certainly know when something is wrong, and resist being loaded up for market. I always felt a slight sense of guilt, particularly about my favourite cows like Rainbow, a mostly black Friesian. She had a distinguishing white ring around her tail.

Once loaded, the lorry drove out of the yard entrance and went up the hill heading for Exeter and the cattle market. About two hours later, Dad and I would follow the narrow road to Exeter, down the hill past the Royal Oak pub at the bottom of the hill, and turn right towards Marsh Barton, where the old market once stood.

The principal auctioneers were called Husseys, and as far as I know they are still in business today. At eleven o'clock the sale would begin. Cattle were paraded in the ring, now with lot numbers stuck on their backs, and the bidding would commence.

The saddest part of the whole event was to see and hear the calves left after lunch, for they were mostly the unwanted ones. The sheep were kept in pens out in the open part of the market, usually about six or eight to a pen. If you thought human beings could be cruel to one another, watch a pen of sheep. If one of their number has a disability the others will kick it into a corner.

The sale over, Dad would go to the office and collect his cheque, assuming his sheep had met their reserve price, then it was back to town and a visit to our favourite fish and chip shop.

The twin Morris Oxfords

Today in 2020 most of us are very security conscious.

It was very different in my younger years. One day Dad drove to market as usual, parked our almond green Morris Oxford in the car park, and went into the market to gauge the trading, as it could vary a bit from week to week. Having completed the business he had to do and met some of his business contacts, he walked back to the car park, opened the car door, put the key in the ignition and drove home.

Not long afterwards there was a phone call from another farmer who had also been at the market and he enquired why Dad had driven off in his car, an identical almond green Morris Oxford. The only difference was the registration number. It is amazing how lax security was in those days – door lock and ignition keys were all the same!

The farmhouse

The house itself had been built over a long period of time, beginning in the late 18th century and ending in the early 20th century. The oldest part was on the right-hand end as you viewed the house from the front. Our house was one which featured two front doors, as the newer part on the left was remote from the earlier part.

Farm Barton had 17 rooms in total, though you would not have liked to live in some of them. The upstairs rooms in the old part of the house we called the rag rooms. They smelled musty and neglected. The floors were unsafe, and the ceilings sagged. Even when a new owner had repaired the floors, they still sloped, which was common in those days. One room, on the very end of the old part, had a rather strange green light, because the main light that got in through the window was reflected from a grassy bank outside.

Downstairs was the kitchen with what mum called the 'hatch', which was sometimes left open on warm summer days. We had two stoves, an Aga, put in in 1952, and a gas stove which was most likely made in the 1920s. In summer mum would not use the Aga as she hated it and the fumes it gave off; it burned anthracite and was probably emitting carbon monoxide.

Past the front door and the porch was what we called the dining room, though we seldom dined in there. In reality it was more like what you might call the living room, and it had an open hearth surrounded with brickwork built by Uncle Bern (dad's brother). Above this fireplace was a long row of cupboards he had also made. Two doors led to the back stairs and to Grannie's drawing room, where she had her upright piano.

Crossing the drawing room was another door to a passageway between Grannie's kitchen and the other front door. The final room at that end of the house was Grannie's 'best' room, which had a beautiful view across Dartmoor. It was typically Edwardian, with all her best Wedgwood china and silver on the dresser. Granny died in that room in July 1964.

The floors in the oldest part of the house were stone, which was common in those early times. Stone can feel quite cold, but as we had the Aga in the kitchen, that was not noticeable. The dining room also had a stone floor, but the fire in there kept the cold at bay. Dad would often come in with fallen branches he had found on the farm, and we would put one end in the fire and as the wood burned, we fed the rest towards the flames.

From the time I was born until the mid-1950s, the house was lit by gas mantles or candles. Then in about 1955 electricity came to the farm in the form of a diesel generator, which was a kind of revolution after gas light.

One thing we children enjoyed about the fire was to make toast using Mum's toasting fork. Sometimes she would lay me on the kitchen table and I would stare at the gas light above and listen to it hissing as it burned.

When I was very young Mum would put me to bed by candlelight and sometimes make an image on the wall of a rabbit with her fingers. One night however she woke me to show me that the house wiring had been completed, and in her hand was a lighted bulb on an extension cable. When mains electricity came a couple of years later it did not affect our life anything like as much did the generator had.

Winter on the farm

Living at the top of a very steep hill could be pretty tough at times. The weather would change very quickly from the warmth of high summer to the icy chill of a winter gale. In the winter of 1962/63 the snowdrifts were level with the tops of the hedgerows, which gave us no escape from this white rural prison. It could give Mum and Dad some really practical problems, such as saving newborn lambs which had been born in the night and had been buried in the snow. We also had to get groceries in for the family, and if it was deep we were not able to get to school in Exeter.

Water came from a well, which would freeze, so Mum would melt snow in a pan on top of the Aga to get drinking water.

In April 1963 the headmaster of my school, Mr Jones, had cause to bring me home after school and I remember that he was flabbergasted to see that there was still snow on the ground when it had long gone in town.

Our social life was non-existent. We just had each other at home for company until the freeze-up ended. Eventually, in March, the bus service began again. I can still feel the cold air coming into the bus as I sat on the long bench seat by the open platform at the back. No health and safety in those days!

On one occasion when I had decided to go into Exeter just after we had had heavy snow, I walked down the lane and up the other side of the valley to our nearest bus stop and waited. Presently, I heard the bus coming down the hill. Seeing a large green object coming towards me with its indicator blinking, I put my hand out to stop it. The only problem was, it was a snow plough! Oops, too late to back away from imminent disaster. One example of how your eyes can deceive you.

Cats

As well as our domestic cats, there was a colony of wild felines who lived in the farm buildings. They were quite numerous, and very prolific. Only one of them had a name – he was known to all as Nicholas Thomas. How he got the name I never knew, but he stood out a mile from all the others.

Grandpa or Dad would squeeze what was left of the creamy milk from the milk filters after milking the cows, and Nicholas Thomas and his mates would appear as if from nowhere to lick up this delicious treat. Nicholas was easily distinguished from the others by his tail, which had a kink in it about half way up, caused most likely when it had got slammed in a door. All these cats were dark brown like most wild felines and were comparatively healthy compared to some on a neighbouring farm which suffered with cat flu.

Every now and then, when the colony grew too large, Grandpa would go out with his shotgun and cull some of them, but he never shot Nicholas. Eventually the wild cats disappeared, so I presume Nicholas died of natural causes and that was the end of them.

We also had three domesticated cats, Marmalardo, a ginger and Ciaddy. Now Ciaddy was in need of medical attention, so the vet was summoned. Ciaddy was an innocent little chap who did not have any idea what was about to happen. Miss Walker, the vet, picked him up and put him head first in a wellington boot, exposing his bottom to the world. SNIP SNIP and they were gone! Job well done. Ciaddy was so shocked that he ran as fast as his little legs could carry him down the garden path, through the yard across the road and across the meadow opposite. We did not see him again for about two months.

Bikes

My first bike was not so shiny and not so new; it had been owned by my cousin in Exeter. One fine May morning I was taken to a stretch of road where I could try out my latest acquisition. Having mounted the bike and with a grown up hanging on to it from behind, I began to pedal. Faster and faster I went gaining in confidence as the machine gained speed, until I realised that they had let go. I struggling to maintain my equilibrium but it was no good, and I was thrown into a ditch and a clump of stinging nettles. It taught me a good lesson, which is that stinging nettles sting!

My next bicycle was a lot bigger, a full size one, bought from new from a shop called Pyles (good name, I thought, for a bike shop). The problem was that where we lived the place was so hilly that I had to push it most of the time. Although it had gears there were none low enough to make much difference, so I had to push it for two thirds of the way home and did not save more than 10 minutes. In the end It was sold to my brother-in-law in about 1974.

That was not the end of my relationship with bikes. In about 1968 my younger sister Chris bought an NSU scooter, a real Mod's bike. Chris did not know how to ride it, so I had the job of showing her how you changed gear. To me it was not a significant problem as you just went one down or two up. You banked when you cornered, except when you were in a field. Most of our fields were sloping, which can make a difference, so for some people that might be a hard thing to do.

After a couple of circuits it was plain sailing to me, and as people say, 'the rest was history'.

The motorbike would have been fine but for the same old problem of steep hills. Once you were down at the bottom of the hill it did not matter how much throttle you gave it, it just would not pull. We found that the piston rings were worn, so that bike just would not go up a slope on a gradient of more than say one in 30. On the level it was not too bad, but where we lived it was a dead loss. I don't know what happened to it in the end as I went to Plymouth for a job at the TV factory.

Holidays

As a young family we did manage to get time away from the farm and go on a proper holiday in a place which was completely different from our home environment. These holidays took place in the mid-50s, so we must have been very young. Our breaks from the agricultural routine did not happen every year by any means, as finding someone who was able to deal with the twice-daily chore of milking and look after the sheep was not easy. Grampa could milk the cows when we were young, but this job usually fell to Uncle Bern, Dad's brother.

Our holidays were always to Cornwall, which was the logical choice as Grannie's brother Wilf had a chalet bungalow at Cannons Town near Hayle. The big day would arrive and mum, dad and we three children would pile into our little Morris 8

(ETA 497) and off we would go. The journey seemed endless to us kids as Exeter to Penzance is 112 miles (180km approx.) 'Are we there yet Daddy?' was a frequently asked question. 'No,' came the reply, 'we're only at the treacle mines at Sticklepath, which is just before Okehampton.'

The roads then were very bad. We had tarmac in Devon, but at the far end of Cornwall they were still just gravel and dust, which in summer would be difficult. The traffic jams were long also, with many coaches of various colours taking other holidaymakers.

Our first holiday in Uncle Wilf's bungalow was marred when my older sister Ruth developed appendicitis during the drive down. I was too young to understand the gravity of the situation. We stopped at Bodmin and sought a doctor, who sent us on to Hayle Hospital where Ruth had her appendix removed, but it spoilt our holiday in this magical part of the country.

Eventually we saw the china clay tips at St Austell. These mountains of spoil were near our journey's end, which was a relief as mum and dad were frantic now with Ruth's condition. We finally got to Hayle, where the hospital staff took over.

There were several more holidays in Cornwall. We stayed at Cannon's Town again, but this time we stayed with a lady called Mrs. Bennett, who lived near Uncle Wilf's bungalow. On this occasion Ruth was well, which meant we could really enjoy the seaside, which is what people go to Cornwall for. Our favourite beach was Lelant, which is very wide and the sand is soft. We also used to visit Hayle beach, Carbis Bay and others.

One of Cornwall's most iconic features is St Michael's Mount. Even today I can see it in my mind's eye, peeping out through the hedgerows as I approach St Erth station when I am travelling down on the train. It really is magical. We visited the Mount on many occasions, walking across the causeway at low tide or catching the ferry at other times.

In the early years there used to be an old shipwreck in Mounts Bay that was being cut up for scrap; the men doing the job would go out there on an army DUKW, a six-wheel-drive amphibious modification of the 2½-ton CCKW trucks used by the US military during World War II and the Korean War. The DUKW was used for the transportation of goods and troops over land and water.

The last holiday I remember going on as a family was in 1964 when my older sisters did not come with us, so we just took Mary, who must have been about eight years old. The accommodation was our neighbour's green caravan, which he had towed down there earlier. The caravan met with a sad end once it was back at home on the neighbour's farm when he used it to keep a ram away from his flock of ewes. The ram decided it did not like its confinement, and butted its way to freedom through the caravan's wall!

In 1968 Dad and I did a journey around the coast of Britain in our VW Beetle. We spent a week travelling up the east coast through East Anglia, Yorkshire, Northumbria and the east of Scotland, then down the west coast to Glasgow, where the Erskine suspension bridge was still being built, then down through Gretna Green and the English Lake District. It was a very enjoyable experience as we did some camping as well as staying at a few inns and boarding houses along the way.

I remember the trains that we saw on a trip to Dawlish. Some of those that ran on the front there had a mixture of different colour carriages, from the days when they were private companies, eg red for LNES, green for Southern Railways and GWR (Great Western Railways, affectionately known as God's Wonderful Railway).

Other holidays I had were one to France when I was 13. We stayed at a convent school near Dieppe in Normandy, visited Paris and the Eiffel Tower and went to Le Havre where we saw the ship *La France* in port. I was amazed at its size. In 1992 I went with a friend to Florida.

CHAPTER 3

Village Life

❖ ❖ ❖

The Village Hall

The old village school closed around the time I was born, and the children were transferred to other schools in the district. My earliest recollection of the village hall was when the Coronation of Queen Elizabeth II took place in June 1953. The hall has undergone many changes since then, the most noticeable being the removal of a partition which had allowed for two classrooms. Some time later an extension to the west end of the old building meant more room for patrons.

The hall's diary was usually full as it was the scene

for many kinds of events, the most popular being the annual pantomime, along with whist drives, dances, jumble sales etc. When I was a little lad I would be taken to see the pantomime at Christmas and the children's Christmas party. I thought the pantomimes were far too long (and still do). All the ladies of the village would work very hard to lay on a special tea for the kids, and as at the school, there would follow party games.

From time to time there would be a village 'hop', but I was not allowed to attend these until I was about 12. We also had a kind of youth club, but I found that it was a bit half-hearted. We took our record player over there, which did make it a bit more interesting as there was music to dance to – this was the era of Merseybeat and the Beatles. The dances were often provided by a local band, usually with 4-6 players who mostly came out from Exeter. One or two were particularly awful, but there were some that were really good to dance to. I met a lot of the local girls and got to know them quite well, but I did not make a lot of progress there, probably due to the hearing loss which was beginning to afflict me.

The hall today is a far cry from the little tin shack that had stood where the village bus shelter is now. It has a good stage and a green room, and my sister Ruth tells me that the kitchen and toilet block have now been upgraded.

A lot of what I saw in our town in those years was drab and tumbledown with few signs of rebuilding. Exeter's High Street was the only evidence that progress was being made in the recovery from the war with new shops and a new look.

Sports Day

During the summer the village would have a sports day. This I liked because I was very good at the 100 yards (not metres) sprint! It was a good way to end my school career.

The event would be held in a local farmer's field opposite the village shop. There would be all the usual competitions and races for the children, and the tug of war amongst two teams of local farmers or anyone who thought they were strong enough to overcome the opposition.

There was a skittle alley which I know was still in use only ten years ago when I went out to Whitestone for the afternoon by chance and discovered they still held a fete there. That was in about 2004.

Looking back at the village hall itself, the original one was built of corrugated iron and was so small we used to say that when you walked in the door you would scrape your nose on the opposite wall!

In winter it was freezing cold and the walls ran with condensation, a perfect breeding ground for infections. It was very similar to the hall depicted in the film 'Cider with Rosie.' which was set in 1920s Gloucestershire. Eventually in the early 1950s it was demolished and socials thereafter were held in what had been the village school.

When I was older, my sisters and I were allowed to go to the youth club there. It was a very tame affair compared to these days. Later our parents said we could attend dances too. This was the place where I met other girls outside the family for the first time.

There cannot be anything more beautiful than a harvest moon, something which I probably became aware of in my mid-teens. They are a wonder to behold and have an atmosphere all of their own. But harvest moons had to be put on hold when I left the farm.

Going to pantomimes

In the mid-1950s when I was a lad of about eight years of age, my sisters and I were often taken to the pantomime and other productions at Exeter's Theatre Royal. The pantomimes were all the traditional ones such as Jack in the Beanstalk. Other shows were mostly Gilbert & Sullivan comic operas like The Mikado and The Pirates of Penzance. As Uncle Lennard and Auntie Edith were both involved in these performances – my uncle was the producer – we often got in free to them.

There would be treats too like peppermint creams, which we loved, but they could not have done our teeth much good. One panto was Dick Whittington. During the performance the cat, played by an acrobat on a trapeze wire, swung from the stage right into our box and it so frightened my sister Ruth that she hid under her seat till the end of the show!

The theatre in London Inn Square had a long history, including two major fires with the loss of many lives. As a consequence, all theatres from then on had to install a fire curtain between the stage and the auditorium. By 1961 audiences were in decline because television had got established, so the impresario Clarkson Rose sold out to an insurance company, who promptly demolished it in 1962.

That really broke my heart. It was such a wonderful place to go, but money talks. Exeter now has the Northcott Theatre on the university campus, but that can never match the atmosphere of the old theatre in the centre of the city which was very much in the Victorian style.

St Catherine's Church

There had been a place of worship in our village since Saxon times, when it would have probably have been open to the elements, with a thatched roof. That would have been replaced with a stone building by the Normans when they came to Britain in the 11th century. St Catherine's was not in the centre of the village but at some distance away on the hill near to where our family home was. As the church was visible from out at sea, it was allowed to fly the white ensign (originally a red cross on a white background.)

Upon entering the building through the outside door there was the porch, and to its left you could see notices related to church matters. On the right of the porch there were the village stocks, which would have been used up until Victorian times. Church porches like ours could be used as places of refuge in days gone by.

The next door led into the main part of the building. On your left were pews and if you looked further there was the font and a door to the belfry. Looking up you could see the minstrels' gallery, most of which was removed many years ago and replaced by the organ, which is still used today. At one time it was pumped by hand by my cousin Richard, who was paid two shillings and sixpence per service.

In front of the organ was our family pew. Looking to the right were more pews and at the far right were the choir stalls, then the altar. Opposite them were some small windows which were glazed with green glass.

In front of that were the lectern and the pulpit. Then we come to the Lady Chapel, the lightest part of the church. At the back of that was a large window with mostly clear glass, but at the top of were four panes of vividly coloured glass which I really loved, because when you went there at 11 am on a bright day they projected such wonderful colours on the floor. The stained glass at the top of the window cast bright colours on the floor: amber, yellow, scarlet, green and cobalt blue.

Another thing about the Lady Chapel was that to the right when you were standing in the chapel and looking to your right there in the pillar was a squint hole which allowed a view of the altar.

Beyond the font there was a small door that led to the belfry. The tower had a peal of six bells, from treble to tenor. I do not know when they were hung there, but they had always been there since my lifetime. When I joined the team of ringers at the age of 12 or thereabouts, the members of the ringers were mostly older than me, so I was mixing with ringers of all ages, and they taught me the rudiments of ringing. On the wall above the little door that accessed the tower was a list of peal changes which was a defined sequence for us to follow, e.g. first to fourth, second to fifth and so on. Halfway up each rope was a fluffy part called the 'sally' which you gripped to start the bell moving. You began to pull on the sally until the bell was 'set in', which meant it was ready for ringing. Hopefully you got into the correct sequence with the other ringers, and joined in a pattern of chimes which gradually changed – for example first to fourth, then third to fifth and so on as called by the captain. The most difficult thing about the peal was setting down at the end of it. An inexperienced ringer might not set the bell in at just the right moment and it would go on ringing.

It was very important for the ringers to keep their feet in the same spot. one ringer moved his foot and caught it in the end of the rope and was pulled up by the weight of the bell, giving him a sprained ankle!

From time to time local parishes would hold bell-ringing competitions, and these could go on all day.

If you live next to a church these can get on your nerves. But it was a good experience for me.

CHAPTER 4

Learning challenges

Idid not find school easy because of the learning challenges caused by my poor sight and hearing. Because my hearing was failing slightly, I often missed vital information which might have enabled me to participate in some events and projects. For example, the school started a musical appreciation class in which each pupil chose a piece of music, usually from a 12-inch vinyl record. Because my hearing was impaired I failed to understand that what was being discussed included a choice for me. I missed out, and that was a theme which would occur again and again in later life. Looking back on it all now, I have begun to understand the severity of my disability, as we usually meet our friends in noisy, crowded situations.

When I was 14, I was sent up to senior class, where we had a very tempestuous master. He was very irritable and, in my opinion, not fit to teach disabled children. This experience caused me to miss school. On one occasion I went into school and while nobody was looking I sneaked down the back lane into Denning Road, then back to Whitestone, where I hid in the church till teatime.

Eventually the demon deputy headmaster was sacked, or transferred to another place in the education system. I was so shocked by the incident of the boy being hit so hard because his disability prevented him from doing what he had been asked to do that I told mum and dad, who had a friend in the village who was one of the school governors.

The end of term came and the whole affair was whitewashed, with plenty of leaving presents, and life for me and many other pupils at St. David's hill improved dramatically.

There were good times at school as well. The excitement would build during the afternoon as the sun sank low, and lessons would be forgotten.

Christmas

Christmas was a happy time. There would be carols at either St David's church or at St. Michael's Roman Catholic Church, which was next to our school. These places were always freezing cold, but that was compensated for by some funny distractions such as one time when the curate was approaching the altar during the most solemn part of the service. Just as he reached the alter steps, he tripped on his cassock and went flying. That raised such a laugh that my girlfriend wet herself with hysterics.

Later we would all troop into the dining room for Christmas tea, with plenty of jelly and ice cream. Then Father Christmas would appear pulling a large handcart laden with presents. The older ones all knew it was really Colin Harris, whose duties at school included being Scout leader and boot and shoe repairer, amongst other things. The presents were distributed, then we usually had some entertainment of some kind.

At midsummer the scouts and guides went on camp. I was not involved in that, but their absence made it very quiet in school so that lessons were quite informal.

The gym

Our gym was a place of fear for me at certain times of the week, when we had to do PE with the demon deputy headmaster. The building itself was quite innocuous, built in the early 20th century I presume. It had four windows, rounded at the top, and one end, the one with the climbing bars, was rather dark. The other end had a balcony, which had on it the school's baroque pipe organ played by Mr Selby, who was blind.

Under the balcony was stored the gym's

equipment, the source of my fear. It was not just me who dreaded PE on Tuesday afternoons. For one lad it was far worse as the demon PE master would thump this lad on his back if he could not perform the tasks asked of him. Jumping a long skipping rope for example was one of the things he just did not have sufficient co-ordination for.

Earlier in my schooling we did as juniors, have musical appreciation classes, and singing with Amey Farnworth, I can recall one song called 'London's Burning' which we had to sing in relays.

The great escape

Every so often, one of the pupils at the school would go missing. I have already mentioned that when I was about ten or eleven I was in fear of the PE lesson on that day and bunked off home to Whitestone and after wandering around the fields, went and hid in St. Catherine's Church. I must have had a wristwatch as I knew when the school bus was due, so I could make my entrance home just after it had gone.

Boarding at school

Later, when I was about twelve, the school staff thought it might be good for me if I became a boarder. To me that was compounding the problems I had with the place.

I began as a live-in pupil at the beginning of the school year that September. At first it did not seem too bad. There was the novelty of teatime, then not having to go back to class after playtime.

There was the new experience of the 'dorm' (senior boys slept in a room with about ten beds). We were usually rounded up by Mr Harris at about 10.15 for bed at 10.30, then lights out. We would lie in bed for what seemed quite a while, listening to 'Lux' (Radio Luxembourg) if any of us had a tranny, and we were soon fast asleep.

Right from an early age sleep was not easy for me. I would lie there feeling restless and wait for the torch that would shine in through the nearest window from the fire escape outside, then I would finally succumb.

When the novelty of being a boarder wore off about two months later I began to understand why the others called this school 'the prison.' We were never let out of the building at night, even under supervision. On one occasion can I remember us marching in a crocodile to the swimming baths for a dip, but it seemed so restricting.

Then one evening I had had enough of being institutionalised. As before, I escaped. Running down the back lane through the back gates which the staff had forgotten to lock, I was free at last. With great speed I ran across the Iron Bridge which ran from St. David's Hill to the junction with Paul Street and North Street. At the top of North Street I turned right into High Street, past British Home Stores and down Fore Street Hill. It was there that one of the masters (not the demon deputy head but another one) made a grab for my arm, but such was my determination to get away that he tore my sleeve and I made my exit from this pursuit down some steps to Exe Bridge and home.

Most of the other escapees were caught right away, but I prided myself in that I got home, never again to be a boarder at that school or any other school. It is a sad indictment of any educational establishment when the pupils regard themselves as prisoners.

Today there is a new school for children with little or no sight at Countess Weir. They return home every weekend where possible, which must be so much better for their wellbeing. Not only that, today they get far more support with their learning needs.

Nightmares

The experience of being in a class run by such a volatile master, who also took me for PE lessons, had a devastating effect on my confidence. For many years after I left school I would have nightmares in which I was pleading for dad to take me away from the school. The weird thing about the bad dreams was that I was the age at which the dreams occurred, which was not until I was around 37. I often wonder what a psychologist might have made of that.

In July 1964 I left St David's Hill for good, but the nightmares still persisted. My future workwise was still uncertain, but from the age of 11 my main interest had been in electronics and TV servicing or engineering. I had a fascination with television and how it worked, particularly the possibility of colour. This was in back 1959, so I would have to wait until 1967 before I would see colour for the first time while living at the college in Birmingham.

An encouraging teacher

There was one member of school teaching staff who had a more encouraging approach to my plight – Mr Neal. He took me under his wing for the last two years of my schooling. He was a BSc and knew of my interest in television engineering. One morning during one of his classes we were scratching patterns on old blank 16mm filmstock so we could see the effect when it was run through the school projector.

During this lesson the conversation turned to videotape, which was then a new medium. Mr Neal explained to the class that like sound, pictures could be recorded on magnetic tape, and it could be edited, though that process was still difficult to carry out. I asked him about the prospects for recording colour pictures and he told me he had seen colour when he went to New York. This really impressed me, and the other pupils in the class were agog with the idea.

Attitudes and styles

When I was born, attitudes and opinions were very different from today. My parents, who were born in the early part of the 20th century, were of course influenced by their parents. A world war, then the roaring twenties, then a massive crash in the economy, moulded their views on behaviour and everything they did.

Mum, who stood about 5ft 6ins tall, was slightly plump and had a rather sad persona, which influenced us children during our growing up.

Dad was about 5ft 10 ins tall and was of slim build, a family characteristic, but did hard manual work all of his life and had a rather dry sense of humour, which was more endearing to us children than to mother.

In the early days when my sisters and I were young

we were expected to be little versions of our parents. We were not expected to get out of line when it came to dress style and fashion, as can happen today. Our clothes were quite sober, my hairstyle had to be "short back and sides". It was definitely a case of "Get your hair cut!" if my hair was beginning to look more than a No. 1 cut, even when I was going to college in Birmingham in 1966.

The dress code of the stars was sober too. The Beatles, the Stones, Freddie and the Dreamers and others were the same. Recently David Bowie died, aged 69. He was one who revolutionised attitudes to dress, style and social attitudes. He changed his hair colour from white to red and was responsible for glam rock.

He also changed people's views on sexuality. In 1966 it was still a crime to be gay, punishable with prison, but the law was changed. Now it is considered "cool" to be in a gay relationship, though still frowned on by some in society, but the momentum is still going that way. We are now all individuals, free to set our own identity and no longer pompous stuffed shirts.

CHAPTER 5

The Swinging Sixties

❖ ⇥ ⊷ ⊶ ⇤ ❖

Flying around Exeter

In 1964 I turned 16 and felt very grown up. I wanted to spread my wings and see more than dung heaps and sheep. I had heard from my big sister that if you went into Exeter and walked up Fore Street hill, half way up was a shopping arcade, and at the far end there was a coffee bar called El Zamba (the name has no meaning in Spanish.) Going in there felt like a dare, so I did so.

There I became acquainted with all sorts of people, many of whom it would have been better not to know. The atmosphere was mostly calm, but the place did have a bit of a reputation. You could get almost anything there, not just frothy coffee and sandwiches.

One thing they had was a juke box, a Seeburg 222. It was unique for its day as it was a stereo one, unheard of at that time. Stereo was rare even in domestic equipment, let alone in hi-fi. All the records were 45 rpm and in mono. The first songs I heard played on it were 'I Could Easily Fall' by Cliff Richard, 'Cast Your Fate To The Wind' by Sounds Orchestral and 'You've Lost That Loving Feeling' by the Righteous Brothers.

So impressed was I that I resolved to own a Seeburg 222 one day. That wish has now come true.

Fashion and politics

The 1960s were the foundation of my adult life. People in public life like Jean Shrimpton, Mary Quant and Twiggy had such high profiles that you couldn't miss them, particularly in the later years of that decade.

As for the fashions, the girls were in mini-skirts that went almost to the top, while the boys just wore jeans, later flairs, and the bikers among them wore leather jackets. The transport of the young then could be dad's borrowed car, or if you were lucky you had a bike, otherwise it was Shanks's pony. My drum teacher once asked me if I could remember the 60s. Remember them? I can still smell them and taste them!

Dad was a member of the local conservatives in the village, and around the end of the 1950s he tried to get me interested in politics. To do this he took me along to the village hall, which was our local polling station, and explained the process and the reason for it. His job was to assist the other clerks during their stint that morning. I did not really understand too clearly at the time, but Mr Macmillan won the election and became Prime Minister and the Conservatives got into power. At the next election in 1963 the Conservatives won again, but with a new leader, Alec Douglas Home.

This was the time of the Profumo affair, in which John Profumo, the Secretary of State for War, was compromised by his relationship with a good-time girl called Christine Keeler who was also linked to a Russian spy. He was forced to resign when he was found to have lied to the House of Commons about it. There was also the Cuba crisis in which the Russians were found to be transporting nuclear weapons to that Caribbean island off the coast of USA, which got everyone very worried, but the thing that really woke me up was the arrival of The Beatles!

I was 14 years old, so this could not have happened at a better time. It was just before Christmas and the first snow was falling outside, and Mum had pulled back the curtains, which were made out of blankets dyed black, a leftover from the war. We had our first 4-speed record changer, a Dansette, so we were ready to go. Over the next few years we built up a good record collection, including Oklahoma, South Pacific and numerous others in addition to the 7-inch pop singles. In later years I collected more recordings of music by Beethoven, Mozart etc.

Radio and TV

Then there was the radio. My first portable radio was a birthday present from mum and dad and was called a Sky Leader, very common at the time. The service then was BBC only. We just had the Light Programme, Network 3 (classical) and the Home Service. Pirate radio was still a couple of years away but it finally happened in about 1964.

In 1963 That Was the Week That Was, or TW3, was born. The old stuffy style of BBC TV was brushed away by satirical programmes like this which began to hit our 17-inch screen. Thus was my interest in British politics established. That programme went out late on Saturday evening after Match of the Day. Its cast was made up of university graduates, including David Frost, Willie Rushton and Bernard Levin. Millicent Martin sang the title song. Their sketches and political observations definitely changed attitudes in this country, and Sir Alec was not a popular leader. In 1964 Labour won the general election, led by Harold Wilson.

The next piece of electioneering which I took interest in was during May 1970, when Ted Heath got the Tories back into power. By now my understanding of the process was far more developed, so when the political circus came to Exeter I went along to the civic hall in Queen Street to hear what Mr Heath had to say. The advice I got from other members of the audience was that you should stand to either the left or right of the hall, according to your political views.

After we had waited for 10 minutes or so, Ted Heath walked on stage accompanied by stripper music!

Later, in 1979, came the big bombshell. Mrs. Thatcher was elected, defeating the last Labour administration after rampant inflation. It led to us losing our farmhouse, but we were able to save the land.

My favourite programme on the BBC in the 60s was Pick of the Pops on Sunday afternoon with Alan 'Fluff' Freeman, and the first song I can remember him playing was Pictures of Matchstick Men by Status Quo.

Early television was rather dull as most programmes went out live, but this led to some strange things happening like when a comic named Charlie Drake was meant to dive through a window, but he knocked himself out in the process and so the BBC just faded the scene out, giving us an apology. Charlie had a fractured skull and was unconscious for three days. He was not able to return to work for two years. Other live shows were less troubled, like Hancock's Half Hour. I can't recall any accidents like the Charlie Drake one happening during Hancock.

Gradually, once tele-recording and videotape got better all the mistakes were edited out and TV was more like today and less no longer unpredictable.

CHAPTER 6

College days

❧ ⸺•⸻•⸺ ☙

A t the age of 16, with school behind me, I began a period of 18 months at home while Dad worked out what he could do to help me learn more about the agriculture business. It would not be easy, as I did not have farming in my heart. All I could think of was electronics and related matters.

In the end my immediate future was decided by a social worker for the blind, Olive Wakeham, who suggested that I should go away to Queen Alexandra College in Birmingham for training in light precision engineering. The first trip to Birmingham, in November 1965, was for me to be interviewed by the principal of the college, Mr Cannon, and I was taken in my cousin John's Wolseley 6/90. When January 1966 came around, mum and I again travelled there in John's car.

What a journey that was. The route was mostly on A roads, as at that time the M5 had only come south as far as Tewkesbury. We set off at about 10 in the morning but did not get to Tewkesbury till about 2.30. The last 40 miles or so when we joined the new motorway were amazing, as John got the 6/90 up to 110 mph.

We got to the college about three in the afternoon, the time I was to check in. I definitely felt like the new boy. Soon after getting there, a passing student kicked me in the shins, which upset me a bit. Months later I learned that that character had cheated in one of his engineering tests, and that had the right psychological effect for me.

Before going into the engineering workshop I had to be assessed. We had to perform simple tests to assess our manual dexterity. These done, I began the course proper with the instructor, Mr Jago. I was taught the use of capstan lathes with all the required tools (there was no automation there.)

Machines in open industry were already converting to numeric control, so our course was already becoming out of date.

The long journey to college

Subsequent journeys from home to the college were made by train or long-distance coach. The coach would leave Exeter coach station at about 10.30 and take virtually all day. The route was Exeter, Cullompton, Wellington, Taunton, Bridgwater, Weston-Super-Mare, then Bristol for a comfort stop. Next was Gloucester and finally Cheltenham for the three o'clock coach transfer, for which all coaches converged from many parts of the country.

The remainder of the journey was a run of 50 miles into Birmingham. We used to arrive at Digbeth bus station at about 16.30, exhausted by the ride. But it was not over yet as I had to walk from Digbeth, up the hill past the Bullring and the rotunda into New Street and then into Corporation street, where I would catch a number 3 bus to Harborne. Quite a long journey, by any standards.

Nearer to the end of my time in Birmingham I was given a travel warrant so I could travel by train between Exeter Saint David's and Birmingham New Street station. This change shortened the time to about four hours.

The college was run in much the same way as school except it had a slightly more liberal attitude to the students. We were still regarded like big children but there was a stronger emphasis on our responsibilities. Drinking was frowned on, but who could stop us from exploring and finding the pub which we did with ease! That got one or two students into trouble, and one was expelled during my time there.

The food was not really enough, and I can recall feeling very hungry at times. One lad discovered that the orderlies had mistakenly put salt in the sugar bowl and demanded that the matron be called. When the dining room assistant refused, he threw his dinner at the wall and said 'She'll see me NOW!' It had the desired effect!

When I was at the vocational college in Birmingham I met many of the students, and their visual impairments varied dramatically. There were some who I thought that compared to them I had no need to be there at all. Some on the other hand were totally blind and always had been, so for them it was completely natural and was a way of life.

One student, who I will call Danny to protect his identity, was one who had lost his sight through no fault of his own but was learning to adapt to his new situation. After breakfast one morning he told me that one morning his mother came into his bedroom and he asked her to open the curtains, but she had already done so, and he said that he could not see anything.

What had happened was that the previous evening his father had come home and knocked the lad down the stairs, which must have caused some catastrophic injury to his sight which had caused him to be blinded.

The point I am making is that my sight was classified as partial and that possibly it might fail in later life, but this poor lad was plunged into the situation which was through no fault of his own.

That meeting really taught me that you must never take anything for granted, particularly your sight.

A murder trial

As students studying at the college in Birmingham we were bound by law to receive lessons in basic English and have an awareness of the British legal system. In 1966 some of us were taken to Birmingham Assizes to witness the verdict in a high-profile murder case involving an Italian kitchen porter and another kitchen worker who was stabbed to death during an argument. We were seated in the public gallery and had a good view of the courtroom, the judge on the bench etc. The judge put the black cap on his head and pronounced the sentence on the man who had been found guilty saying, 'You have been found guilty of this offence and you will now be taken from this place to a place of execution and hanged by the neck until you be dead, and may God have mercy on your soul.' In the seats in front of us was the man's mother, who began crying when she heard the sentence. The sentence was later commuted to life imprisonment, but the memory of that event has haunted me ever since.

I managed to complete the course. The only comment from Mr Jago in my report was that my effort 'flagged at times', something which was made clearer later in 1972 when I had another ability assessment in Exeter. There it was established that I had to put in three times as much effort as others in order to achieve the same result.

Other machines I learned about were vertical drills, horizontal milling machines, shapers and surface grinders, which I would come across in my first job.

I left the college in March 1967 having gained a certificate in engineering, and some new friends, one of whom I am still in touch with.

Heart trouble

From an early age it had been suspected that I might have a heart murmur, so before I started work it had to be properly investigated. I was taken to Bristol

General Hospital for this. After swallowing a barium meal I had to lie on an X-ray table, where a cannula was inserted in my left arm and some opaque dye was poured in. Then the investigation began.

It was the most frightening experience I had had in my life so far. The surgeon, Mr Barratt, wanted to see heart movement under stimulation, very frightening as it was so violent and prolonged. I could see the monitor above my head and at the same time hear what sounded like a cine camera whirring. I enquired what the noise was and was told that a tele-recording was being made of the procedure, as this was a teaching hospital. So I was a guinea pig too! When it was all over I was sent back to the ward, but my heart rhythm did not settle down till the following day.

Some time later, Mr Barratt came to see me. He informed me that there was no hole, but there was a slight deformity which he could not do anything about.

My first job

Having established that there was no real damage to my heart to be repaired, I was ready for my first job. This was at a company called Centrax in Exeter, which made turbine compressor blades for jet engines. Most of the machines I had been taught about were there, including a line of surface grinders, which were classed as semi-skilled work and were high tolerance. My job was simply to put a chunk of metal in a chuck and press a button. It was noisy, boring work, and seemed quite a comedown after all that training in Birmingham. Surely I was worth more than that? My first pay packet contained £7 10 shillings.

The job at Centrax did not last very long. My next job was at a lawnmower service centre, and the work was similar in nature, so that did not last long either.

Rock bottom

At 25 years old, I felt at rock bottom. After all, I was a young man, still viable, or so I thought, but my self-esteem was being challenged. The doctor in Bridgwater had prescribed anti-depressants, but they did not seem to work. It seemed it would take me a long time to recover my own way.

The problems I was accumulating were mounting up and getting worse. I began to realise the true nature of my lack of social skills, which I should have learned years ago. My friend Peter at work in Bridgwater was 25 and already married with a son of 18 months, and here was I still in the same position as of a teenager. It was like a rocking chair, marking time while my life was at a standstill, seeking relief rather than going out and trying again. That was when I would have thoughts of seeking some advice about these things.

Back to the farm

I returned to work for my Uncle Bern (dad's brother) on the other family farm. Agriculture was now more modern, and tractors were more powerful than the ones I knew when I was five years or so. However we did have a Field Marshall on tracks which dated from 1948, which was a bit of a curiosity.

Since 1964 my uncle had put up an egg-laying plant which contained 7,500 laying hens, later expanded to 10,000 birds. My job was only part time, but it seemed preferable to either of my engineering jobs in Exeter. I would go round with a trolley collecting the eggs and then wash and grade them. The work did not pay much, but the hours added up and after all, there was nothing to spend the money on out there in the sticks.

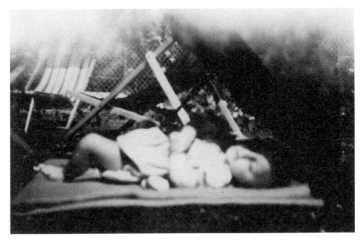

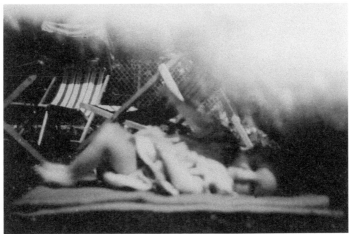

Robert. Auntie Nina's Garden, summer 1948

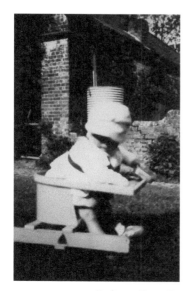 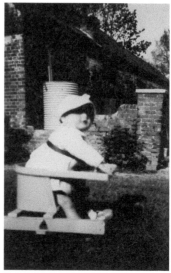

Robert. Farm Barton Garden. 1948

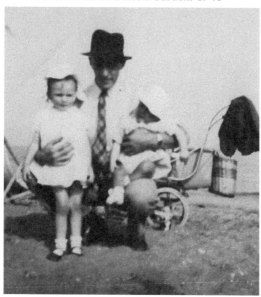

Robert as a baby with Ruth and Dad, summer 1948

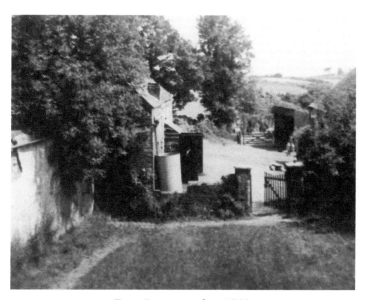

Farm Barton garden. 1950

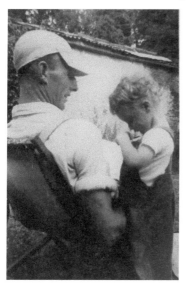

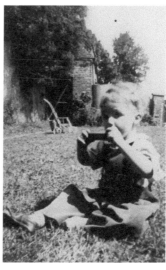

Farm Barton garden. 1950

Robert, 1950,
Farm Barton garden

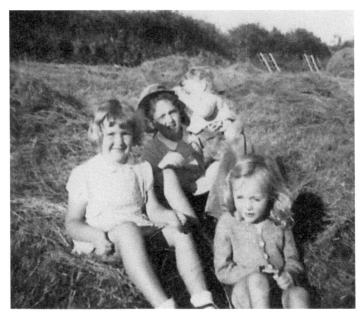

Cousin Jane and Cousin Susan holding
Robert with Ruth, summer 1950

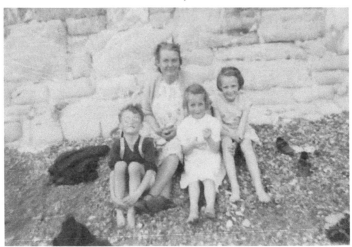

Mum, Ruth, Robert and Christine sitting by the sea wall, Dawlish

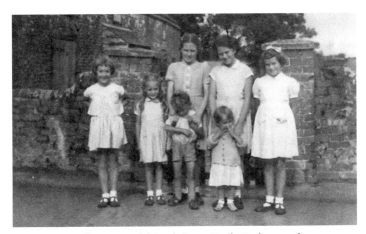

Belle, Sue and friend, Jane, Ruth, Robert and
Christine, Farm Barton, 1951

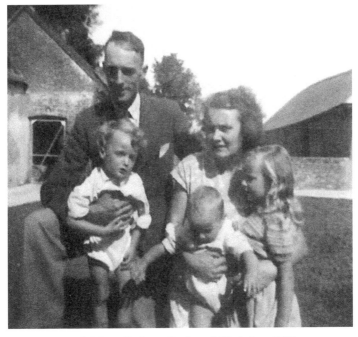

Dad, Mum, Robert, Ruth and Christine, 1951

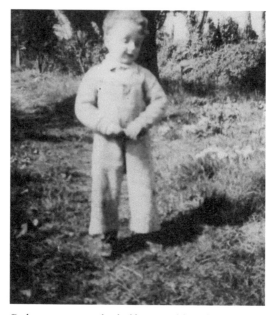

Robert at two and a half years old in the top garden

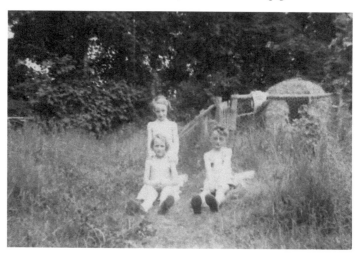

Ruth, Christine and Robert outside the playhouse
made by Mum. Top garden. 1956

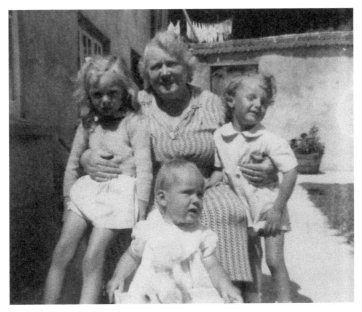

Granny Netherway, Ruth and Robert. Farm Barton Garden. 1951

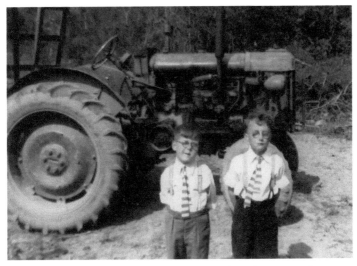

Robert (aged two and a half) and Ruth in the top garden

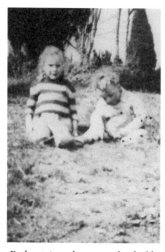

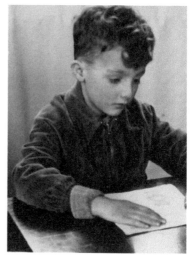

Robert (aged two and a half)
and Ruth in the top garden

Robert aged 7. School 1955

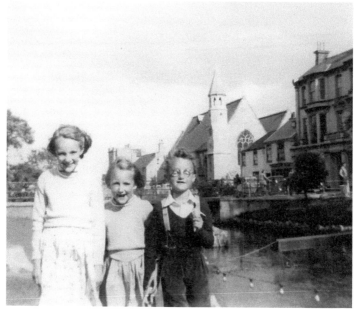

Ruth, Christine and Robert. Dawlish 1955

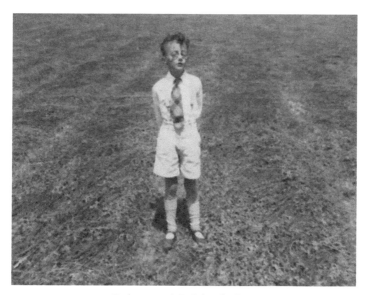

Robert aged 7. School 1955

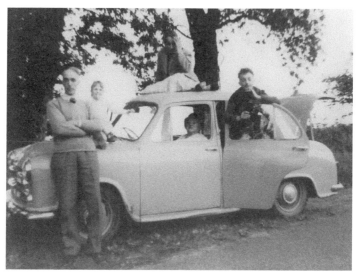

Dad, Mary on bonnet, Christine on car roof, Granny Netherway
in car, Robert leaning over door. Trip out, 1959

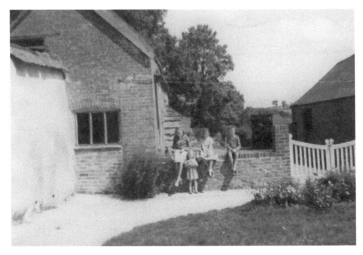

Ruth, Christine and Robert sitting on wall, Mary standing, 1959

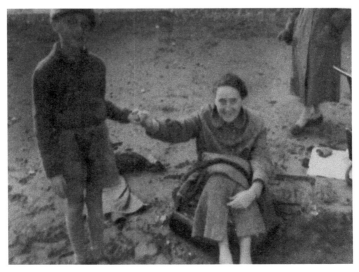

Robert and Auntie Betty, Dawlish beach, 1957

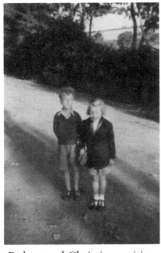

Robert and Christine waiting
for the bus, September 1964

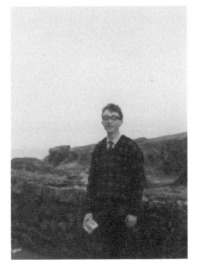

Robert on a trip to Corwall

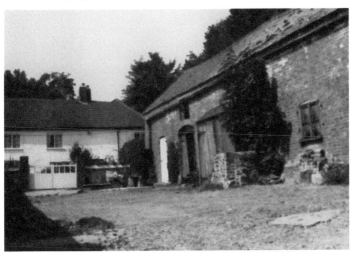

Farm Barton courtyard, 1966

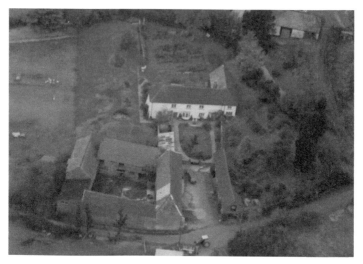

View of Fam Barton house and yard. Date unknown

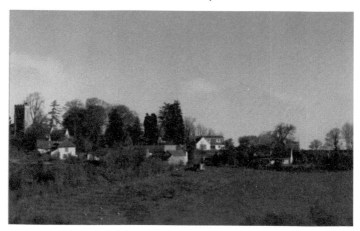

View of Whitestone Church, farmhouse and buildings. Dad's
bungalow on the right

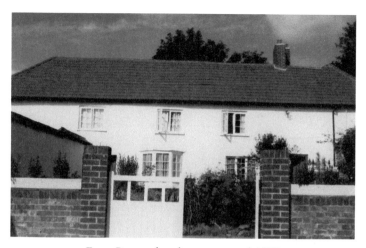

Farm Barton farmhouse, around 1970

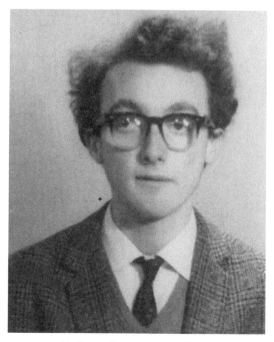

Robert's first passport photo

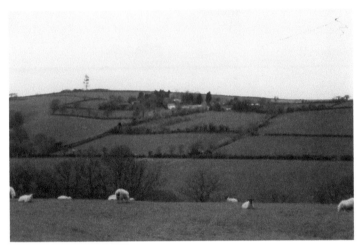

View of Farm Barton from Whitestone village

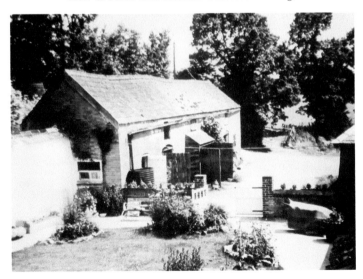

Farm Barton

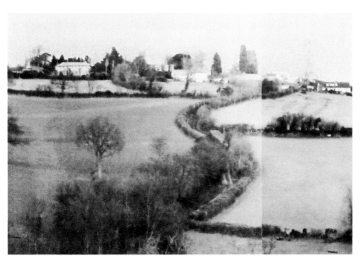

Farm Barton, circa 1966

CHAPTER 7

Training for a career

✦❖✦

While I was working on the farm I started an evening class at Exeter college studying a City & Guilds course in radio and television servicing. Being with other like-minded students really improved my morale and sense of purpose. In those days there was no multiple choice, just a written answer. In the class there was one lad who noticed that my sight was not 100 percent and started showing off just to make me feel small, but he did not turn up for the exam! The course completed, I sat the exam and passed both parts with a credit and a pass.

Colour TV had started on BBC2 the previous year and was being extended to the other two channels, so I was very keen to try hard and get a job in that field. Time went on, and eventually in January 1970 I got a job at Rank Bush Murphy in Plymouth, a huge place employing over 2,000 people. I was engaged as a prototype technician, which boosted my confidence a bit. From the first day I could tell the evening classes had paid off as my knowledge was already better than that of some of the others in my group.

INSTRUCTOR: What is the bandwidth of a standard 625-line pal signal?

ANSWER: DC to 6Mhz.

INSTRUCTOR: What is the frequency of a PAL colour sub-carrier?

ANSWER: 4.43361875.

GOT IT! and so on.

Unfortunately my time at Bush was cut short when it was discovered that I could not see the coloured value rings on a ¼ watt resistor. I felt absolutely gutted, so I went home again.

In the summer of 1971 there came another engineering job, at Bridgwater in Somerset. I had been advised by the DRO (Disability Resettlement Officer) that it was soul-destroying work. but it paid very well. This was another large factory, this one manufacturing electric water pumps for central heating systems. We were producing over 3,000 of these units per day.

Like the first job at Centrax in Exeter it turned out to be boring, tedious work, just as the DRO had predicted. The pay there though was very good for the times and I would often take home £34 per week, which enabled me to start saving towards a deposit on a house one day. For a long time I worked in despatch, removing the drain plugs from the motors after they had been pressure tested, but I enjoyed the company of my fellow workers, about 30 of them. Not only that, we were all on the same lunch break.

Then, disaster! I was moved into the main part of the building, where it was noisy, dark and depressing, and, worst of all, on a different lunchtime, so cutting me off from the social contact which I had built up over the previous two years. That was the final blow, the end of another chapter in my working career.

Wherever I had gone to get a job I had been found lodgings. Some were good, others not so good. The last of these was with a nice couple who had retired from farming pigs in a place called Woolavington, which is just north of Bridgwater. Bridgwater is famous only for two things, the carnival, with its colourful floats, and squibbing, and the fair held in September. I did enjoy both of these events as there was little else going on in Somerset.

Slowly, month by month, things began to improve again, and after just over a year I felt much better again, my confidence returning.

At about the same time my older sister Ruth got married to Paul, who came from Lydney in the Forest of Dean. We were having our new bungalow built then to replace our old farmhouse across the road, which was having to be sold. I was very interested in the new start and took many photographs of the construction in progress.

The plan now was to retrain for a different kind of job, so went on a course at Saint Loye's college in Exeter which trained disabled people. Full of hope once again, I passed the tests and did a course in telephony and typing, which was one of the few jobs open to me. That done, the gateway to a life in Bristol awaited me.

My sight gets worse

in the late 1980s I began to notice that my sight was beginning to deteriorate. During a routine eye examination in 1986 the consultant at Bristol Eye Hospital diagnosed glaucoma. A couple of years later I began to get the symptoms of that condition. When looking at a high-contrast image, parts that should appear black or very dark now looked slightly misty. That did not inhibit my behaviour too much, but as time went by it got worse. Reading the printed word became harder as sometimes the print would suddenly get very black, then fade. I noticed too that my writing was fading when I wrote anything with a ball-point pen. The effect was like looking through those transparent bags you get in the supermarket.

I soon began to need help to navigate the streets. People who will help you to get around come in all shapes and sizes. Most of those I meet in the street are anxious to help, and usually do. Now and again I meet one who just grabs my wrist, and without saying a word gives me a quick mobility lesson. Then, there is the one who does ask what you want but does not tell you where the pavement edge is, or walks you off the pavement at an oblique angle so you nearly lose your balance, or worse, twist an ankle. The answer to all this is a guide dog. I have considered this many times but feel that I would not manage the situation well enough to outweigh the disadvantages.

In the 90s, my sister Mary and my brother-in-law thought it might be a good idea if I were to move once again to live near to them, so in 2001 I pulled up my roots and went to live in Cardiff. It seemed like a logical thing to do, but once I got there did not settle. I stayed for two and a half years before I came back to my own side of the Bristol Channel.

CHAPTER 8

Personal issues

❧ ⸱⸱⊶⸱⊷⸱⸱ ❧

The mystery of girls

Having put school and college behind me, and having been busy with work for a while, I did not have any real girlfriends to speak of in my early 20s, just the odd casual friendship with those I had met in the village or in Birmingham. I now felt things should be getting more interesting. After all I had a good job at the pump factory in Bridgwater, and I used to go to the local youth club in the town even if I was at the top of the age range. But the isolation continued, and things were still the same.

There were times when in the evenings after work I would go for walks around the town and see young couples, some younger than me, holding hands or embracing each other. What was this magic formula they shared with one another? Why was it that if I had a conversation with a girl it was always on the "what nice weather we are having" level? It was a mystery to me. After all, I wore the same sort of clothes and my manners for a 25-year-old were reasonably good. I just could not understand why things never worked for me.

My frustration grew and grew, making my blood boil even more than before, and I was worried that I might attack someone one day. Fortunately for me that never happened, though it nearly did a couple of years later.

Living a life of enforced celibacy on top of my sensory deprivation drove me to thoughts of suicide several times as it did not seem to matter where I lived, the problem just would not go away. In 1977 I sought advice from a psychologist who put me through a course of therapy, and at the end of this we had a party where we were watched to see how we interacted with the others. The psychologist's conclusion was that I was a bi-guy, and that I could have "twice as much fun"!

Slowly but surely I began to withdraw, my effort dwindled and I just gave up on myself.

Solitary confinement

The solitary vice is a vicious circle. It reduces your will to go out and try again and at the same time relieve any pressure you are under. Like worry, it is like that rocking chair, it just keeps on rocking. To me it was a kind of solution to my needs, but at the same time it was helping me to avoid facing up to the problem of negotiating with a potential partner whilst coping with partial sight and deafness, and the lack of confidence and the social skills which I should have acquired back in the village. Over the years it became the norm, and I gave up expecting anything to change. This was what led me to despair and thoughts of suicide. Quite often I would ask myself, am I fertile? If I had children, what would they look like? and so on. Other questions included, 'would I be able to support my family?'

Well, now I know some of the answers.

Dreams

We all dream at one time or another during our sleep. While I was young I do not remember dreaming all that much, I would just go out like a light. Suddenly it would be morning and I would be shaken gently by mum, saying 'Come on, time to get up for school.' I can't remember protesting about it at all, so I must have been a very obedient little boy. It was only later when I was aged 11 or 12 that I began to resist getting up for the day of fear at St. David's Hill and all that led to those nightmares.

Fortunately when I did have dreams they were pleasant, the kind you get at puberty. Later on when puberty was past, my dreams would be of happier matters, like our farmhouse and my uncle and aunties' homes. The farmhouse at Pitt Farm where my four cousins lived, Isobel, John, Richard and Beth, was one place where I used to find myself in dreams more than in our own house. I put this down to the fact that our family was rather withdrawn from social activities and there was not much contact compared to our cousins, who were more outgoing than us.

Later still, my dreams would be about times past. Sometimes I would dream about places where I had been living, but they would not manifest themselves until about five years after the time when I had been there. One dream in particular I remember having when I lived in my first flat in 1978-80. I would find myself going to the local shops, and for some reason I would be in the little supermarket nearby.

The dream which was most persistent was, and still is, about the house I lived in from 1985 to 2001. That was in Snowdon Road, here in Fishponds where I live now. About five years after leaving it, I would dream I had returned there and had somehow got in, but was anxious that the new owners would come back and find me there. Later versions of that dream would be cluttered with all the things you collect over 20 years and should have got rid of long ago. My next-door neighbours also featured in the later versions. I wonder if I will have any more dreams about life at Snowdon Road.

Occasionally my dreams are about driving around the narrow lanes from Exeter out to the farm with the BT tower that was built in 1959-60 to carry ITV (Westward Television) from their new studios in Plymouth to the transmitter at Stockland Hill near Honiton. My hope now is that in a few years I shall start dreaming about being the drummer in some big rock band, doing fantastic gigs with appreciative audiences!

Destinations

All through my life I have from time to time wondered if there really is an after-life. The subject is a perplexing one, as theologians will assure us that there is one, but I have my doubts about it. Several times I have been under a general anaesthetic, which renders all the senses inoperative, so I have had absolutely no sense of anything. No sight or hearing, none of the other things that make us aware, particularly time.

On one occasion in 1991 I had to have a fairly major operation for the removal of varicose veins. The procedure must have taken two hours, as the clock in pre-op said 11.30 and the next thing I knew the clock in recovery was reading 1.30 pm. There was absolutely nothing in between those two events.

As the body decays after death there is no brain, ears or eyes to produce any kind of sensation. I have read a lot about the near-death experiences that people claim to have had, but then those people have regained consciousness and returned to life.

However if there really is an afterlife I think I would want to return to the 1970s, for that was the decade of my young adult years. At the beginning of the decade I was 22 years old and being brought up on a farm in rural Devonshire with loving parents, something some kids could never hope for. At the end of that decade I was 32 years old and entering adulthood, and a bit wiser but still full of optimism.

If possible I would want to be able to take side trips to the past, perhaps medieval times. Of course I would only be there in spirit so I could come to no harm. And maybe I could go forward in time to see what we mortals had done to Planet Earth in the intervening years.

My earthly requirements would be a decent motorbike, and to be able to use it where there are no traffic jams and there is decent weather and all the best food. In the evenings I might go to my favourite music venue, where I would find some human comfort after all the isolation from people that I endured whilst living on Planet Earth.

Jesus rose from the dead, and sat on the right hand of God the Father Almighty. If he came to me personally and said 'Bob, it's really good here' I don't think I would worry about it or doubt it.

CHAPTER 9

Riding the air waves

For as long as I can remember I have loved radio – its virtue is that you can hear it wherever you go. My earliest recollection of the 'wireless', as it was known when I was small, was Listen With Mother after lunch, just before mum would lay me down to rest for a while she caught up on her housework. The radio we had, which dad bought in about the late 40s, was a battery-operated one and its batteries did not last very long. I still have that radio now.

We made a big leap into the 1980s when citizens band (CB) came to the United Kingdom From

America. I was reluctant at first to join in with the other CB users as the type of transmission was called amplitude modulation, which caused interference to other broadcasters such as BBC radio and television, but inevitably I got a 'rig' as they were called and used to go out and 'eyeball' other CBers.

Back in the mid-1970s, after leaving the college in Birmingham where I had met my lifelong friend Dave, I learned that he was interested in the idea of doing amateur radio and soon afterwards he had passed the exam, plus the Morse test. The combined exam and Morse test were, I felt, too much all at once, so I waited in the hope that the regulations might become less stringent.

At around the same time in the mid-1970s I met a friend who was planning to build a bungalow. He had bought an old prefab which already had planning permission. The plan was to build the bungalow around it then demolish the prefab from within, and I helped him with the work. It took about three years but we completed it.

In the 1980s I was to meet two other friends who were studying for their radio amateur transmitting licence and by 1990 we had been on several holidays taking the amateur radio equipment with us, once to Lundy island in the Bristol Channel, and another time on the canals in the English Midlands.

Soon after moving into my house in Fishponds at the end of 1984, I set up my CB radio kit and got on the air again.

A few years went by, and bonanza! The Government relaxed the requirements and divided the radio transmitting licence exam into two parts, 'A' and 'B.' This meant I could do the two stages separately and sit the 'B' exam before doing the Morse test. By then Dave had qualified and had his full licence. In 1990 I got my 'ticket', as amateurs call their licence, so I was now G1XTQ. In May the following year, 1991, after much practice on the Morse key, I got my full licence (G 0PDV), which allowed me to surf the world on all frequencies that the Government allows. I was even allowed to transmit television so long as it was not rebroadcasting commercial transmissions like the BBC or ITV.

One of the first contacts if made through CB radio was a lad whose handle was the Artful Dodger, though his real name was Paul. He had a Suzuki 100cc bike and he was very keen to take me on it to go to steam rallies, so I bought a crash helmet which now rests at the back of my sofa as a reminder of all our adventures to places around Bristol. The rides led us various places including Frocester in Gloucestershire and Bleadon near Weston-super-Mare. The longest ride was to Netley Marsh, which is just outside Southampton. I shall never forget that trip as we left Fishponds at 2 pm and were in the showground by 4.15 – an amazing time for a little bike like that one.

The rally had steam rollers, showmen's engines, tractors like the Field Marshal and old cars. Paul was well acquainted with these vintage engines and tractors. I am always glad he took me to see these things as the interest has never left me.

Being able to go on adventures like those bike rides opened up a whole new world for me. It was such a big new experience, although most reasonably well-off young men in the early 80s could do it.

In 2014 I found out about another steam rally at Monmouth and this time my youngest sister Mary and my brother-in-law Jim took me, so the flame was still burning in there.

Computing

Computers have been around since Tommy Flowers developed 'Colossus', which was the first real electronic number cruncher, developed as part of the war effort in the early 1940s. The next step was 'LEO', a commercial machine used by a catering company to calculate their wage bill.

The first computer I encountered was installed in Exeter in about 1960 for an insurance company. We were ushered into the building and given a brief description of what we were about to see, and then came the real thing. Looking through a glass wall from a viewing gallery we could see a lot of gigantic tape streamers looking like pairs of large eyes. There were samples of the tapes for us to examine – the tapes were four inches wide, like early videotape. That was it. We were told by Mr Neal, our science master, that the future for computers was bright. Not many years later that insurance company left Exeter.

My next encounter with the computer was in the mid-1970s when my brother-in-law got a BBC model 'B' which the BBC had had made in order that schoolchildren could learn more about what was going to be required of them when they grew up. It came with a floppy disk drive, and the disks were about 5 or 6 inches in diameter, and could hold only a few kilobytes. Computer core memory was limited to 10K or so. How did we manage in those days?

In about 1992 with one of my amateur radio friends, Mike, I decided to build a home computer. By this time component parts were being made, mostly by Chinese. A box was procured from a local shop called Target Electronics, and then bit by bit we bought the rest, sometimes going to London for the day, where supplies were more plentiful. Floppy drives were still being used but the memory was doubling every 18 months, and the disks themselves were much smaller. By that time my project would have a very respectable specification.

In the meantime I had bought several Sinclair Spectrums, and they taught me the rudiments of writing software. I also bought an Omega 500, then a 1200. These I wanted because the output could be in PAL which is, or should I say was, the TV video standard of that time. With the Omega 1200 and a VCR I could make titles for the camcorder I now owned.

One afternoon in about 1989 TV programmes were interrupted for an important announcement. We were told that a very significant development was to take place, and so the World Wide Web was born, I was intrigued by that news.

Finally, I got into standard computers in the now legendary tower. My project was complete by the end of 1993 and went 'live' in January 1994, and it included a dial-up modem. Today I am using a laptop connected to the internet and my electronic drum kit so I can practise to songs on Youtube. Whatever next?

The discovery that Exeter had an amateur radio club and that I had a new friend with Alan was a relief, as living in Cardiff had been a bit of a nightmare. One of its virtues was that it was only 40 miles from Bristol, which I could visit on a fortnightly basis. Every other Sunday I would catch the train and visit my old haunts such as the Mason's Arms in Stapleton where I knew a lot of people who I felt easy with. During that time living in Exeter the once fortnightly visits to BS16 carried on until I could move back to Bristol permanently, which I did in February 2006.

CHAPTER 10

A home of my own

❧ ⸺•⸺ ❧

When I moved to Bristol in 1978, my new home was a purpose-built flat on the boundary of Fishponds and Downend. It was built in 1973, so it did not have any serious issues with construction, and it had a spacious garden at the back. I thought I had landed on my feet this time and soon re-established my connections there.

By this time my sight was going fairly rapidly. I could still see the essentials and could ride my bike on main roads, but this was more challenging than before and I had several near misses. I decided that I would have to give up bikes and concentrate on my radio hobby, which I did with G 8BSP back in

Devon via a repeater station, G B3WR, which was successful.

2006 was the year I came back to Fishponds in Bristol, which I had got to know before I left my home in Snowdon Road in 2001. Part of the reason for coming back was that my heart was not anywhere else, and still is not. Bristol works for me. and always will. When I came back there were quite a few people living around the neighbourhood who had known me for a number of years, and I was determined to rebuild my relationships with them.

By that time my sight was failing me. Images were now weak and I could only see vague shapes and could not deal with rapid changes, so I was no longer able to ride my bike on the road.

First, I had looked around the estate agents and found a suitable flat to invest my bricks and mortar in. Very soon an agent found a flat that I was able to afford. It had all things that I needed and was on the ground floor. At first I did not know if the service charge would be affordable, but as time went on I felt more comfortable with what was asked.

Housework

Yes, there is housework to do, even in my home. I am not the tidiest of people, but even I like the place to be kept in some kind of order. When I had my first home at a place called Chetwood House, where I lived from March 1978 until October 1982, I found it an easy matter to run a tight ship, if it was just a case of vacuuming the obvious dust and dirt. But some of the smaller stuff like crumbs would get missed and would never get cleaned up. Polishing the furniture was something I did not mind doing, and any visitors that called did not sniff the air and pull a funny face. This was reassuring, as before all this I had wondered if I could manage to look after a homed after growing up with a mother whose attitude was so negative. When I was small she would give me a job to do like painting the window sills and the shutters in the living room at the old house, then because I might make a mess of it she would take over and finish it. This did not lead me to have much confidence when doing jobs around the house. At least when I left home my confidence grew, as I knew it was down to me to judge whether what I had done was satisfactory.

Cooking was rudimentary – no microwaves then, just an electric cooker, a fridge that a friend had lent me and a Belfast sink to do the washing up. I got an old armchair, which was too big for the flat, but beggars can't be choosers. A coffee table followed and so on

Later I felt that where housework was concerned I needed to employ someone to help me to do the cleaning was now essential, so I got an agency to provide a cleaner and shopping guide. That made a big difference. The agency girls would come once a week to take me shopping and do the housework.

A trip to Bordeaux

Now having really arrived, Bristol was my oyster. My contact list was growing fast as I thought it ought to. After the village, which was so limited this felt wonderful. There seemed to be no limit to where and what a chap might do. The link from Dave and his landladies' son Andy led to people at the National Federation of the Blind, and so on.

In 1980 the N.F.B. had links with the Bristol-Bordeaux twinning association and, with two people I met, I spent a week in that city. The visit to Bordeaux was an enjoyable one, I often think of the time when I went there, and how near to Britain it was, but so different in character. The people we met there were most hospitable and we were looked after very well. I met some people from a school for the visually impaired and learned about the French government's policy towards them.

There were the activities at the Bristol settlement too. 1980 was also that royal wedding, and I had a girlfriend for a time. Our dates were centred around going to the pictures as we both loved Mr Bond, 007!

Discovering music

My opinion of the popular music scene of the 1980s was not high. Punk ruled OK, but it was definitely not to my taste, and even in the mid-90s things were not much better. Robbie Williams and Oasis seemed to dominate. But later in life I was able to begin making music myself, something I had always wanted to do. This opened a new and rewarding chapter in my life.

CHAPTER 11

Making music

❧ ⸺•⫘•⸺ ❧

In 2007 I would regularly walk past one of our local pubs, the Portcullis on Fishponds main road, and find I could hear live music coming from upstairs. So without so much of a how do you do I went in, and enquiries established that it was indeed a regular open mic night.

A talent for drumming

Needing to prepare myself for some involvement, I got in touch with an organisation that offered music therapy and some advice. I went to their studio, where a very friendly tutor introduced me to the piano. After only a short while she announced that I would never be a pianist. I knew she was right, as I had dropped out of piano lessons at school. However, she tried me with an assortment of drums and lo and behold she said, 'You have a natural ability - you will be able to pursue drumming.'

After a couple of weeks had gone by, I went back to the Portcullis and joined the open mic club. By that time I had begun drum lessons with Colin Aldridge, who was once the house drummer at the Colston Hall in Bristol, no less. My first lesson was in August 2007, and I still have a tape recording of it. The first year was excruciating, but Colin assured me 'the first ten years will be the worst, then things will get better!' He was right, as in the end I became sufficiently confident to play for the local band Revamp during open mics. The struggle with Colin's lessons, which took me through grade 1 and 2, have been worth it. My estimate of my ability now is between grade 2 and 3. Jerry Osborne, who led the open mic sessions, also gave me lessons for a while.

By the middle of 2008, Colin thought I was ready to sit the exam, which I passed with 69 marks.

At the open mic I met three other budding musicians, Peter (vocals and lead), Paul (rhythm and some vocals) and Jacky (electric bass). After some conversation we started asking ourselves what it would be like to be in a band. My answer to the question was, 'There's only one way to find out – form one'.

By 2009 the band had a name. After a short discussion, Pete's wife Sue suggested 'MLC', which we were informed stood for Mid-Life Crisis! As nobody could think of anything better, that name stuck. We had absolutely no idea what we were in for, especially when we got our first gig at a place called the Fire Engine in St George. What was it like? A NIGHTMARE! the stage was slippery, which meant my kit kept sliding away from me. I did not know that it was best to put the kit on a rubber mat to stop it sliding around.

Gradually we learned to set things up so that life would be easier for us. Soon we began practising at a studio called Limbo One, and things got better – gradually.

At the open mic night I found the band of musical enthusiasts were very welcoming, unlike Exeter where you were expected just to be in the audience and clap where appropriate. Here you were welcome to join in so long as you showed an interest in music and were willing to learn.

The first new friends I made at the Portcullis were Pete Craig, Paul Hutton and Jacky Tipcombe. Pete, who played lead guitar, was the first one I spoke to. He was, and still is, a team leader at work, so I assumed he would be a natural leader of any band. Paul played power chords and Jacky was on bass. When I joined them I was still a beginner as a drummer, so it was to be a long road ahead, but inevitably the question was raised as to whether we could make a band out of our skills and make a go of it. I said to them that there was only one way to find out.

Building up a set list

We found a studio, Limbo One in Kingswood, and went there to make a start on our musical adventure. We all had our favourite songs, so we looked through the song books picked out what we thought were straightforward songs to learn. Among the first songs we attempted were 'Back in the Night' by Dr Feelgood and 'No Matter What' by Badfinger. Gradually we built up our set list until we had 20 songs.

In general the songs we chose were covers of popular numbers brought out in the 70s and 80s. On average it would take about three weeks to learn each one. There were very easy ones like 'The Passenger' by The Pretenders – we got that one nailed in about the time it runs for – and then there were others like 'Dakota' by the Stereophonics, which took around a month of sessions to get right. The set list grew gradually until we had about 20 songs, not quite enough for a full set, but enough for a warm-up band.

Once we had our first gig behind us we decided to keep going and try to get another one. An agent was sought and he booked us for a gig at Yate town park, very near to where Pete lived – that was in the winter of 2010.

The months rolled by from the February of 2011 until the beginning of June. By that time we were practising once a week, but then we doubled the rehearsals to twice a week. The excitement and the tension grew with each day, and it was almost unbearable to the point that the bass player nearly quit, leaving the rest of us with no bassist. The feeling was that with only ten days to go it was all over, nothing was going to happen. But after some soul searching and new T-shirts provided by Jacky, the show was back on the road.

By 2009, we felt sufficiently sure of ourselves to approach an agent and find a festival. We missed the closing date but went on practising for the next year or two until, in late 2010, we were successful in getting our first gig, which was at Yate Music Festival in June 2011. The requirement was that we should play 10 songs. As most songs last for three and a half to four minutes, that would mean we would be on stage for about 35 minutes.

Making musical friends

The next stage of my now-improving social life was moving from the Portcullis in Fishponds to the Portcullis in Staple Hill. This was a disaster, as the car park was non-existent and the band had to play behind an L-shaped alcove which made the acoustics very strange indeed, and the landlord did not appear to like us!

One person who was a great source of encouragement was Rob Davies, a musical instrument demonstrator with a local music shop. Rob, by the nature of his job, was a multi-tasking genius and when you played for him and the band you could feel that you were at the top of your game.

In the latter part of the year two more faces appeared. The first one was Paul (Yogi) Dutfield, another would-be drummer whose skills were also bass and (I understand) power chords, but he wanted to develop his drumming. The second person to join us was a very nice young lady called Karina, who was a vocalist.

Amidst all this activity I was having great trouble trying to hear what the others were talking about 'as being forewarned is to be forearmed.' In recent years however, people who know about the problems I face have become familiar with my needs, just as with ways to wellbeing did.

Last but not least my three most recent friends, who I met in 2017, are Vicky, who has helped me so much with editing this book, Andy (Gibby) lead guitar in the current band Revamp, and Paul Doyle, who plays bass.

The show must go on

Have you heard of Sod's Law? If you haven't, then I am going to tell you about it. It goes like this. You have something very important that you have been working on for months and months, then from out of the blue something happens which could ruin your plans. In my case it was a hernia. For some time I had been getting pain in an embarrassing place, so I went to the doctor, who said 'You've got a hernia.' Now, with only a short while before we were to do the Yate festival, this thing was really killing me. It was so painful, and worst of all I had to keep poking it back into my anatomy. Can you imagine how awkward it must have been?

The show must go on however, so on 'Big Saturday', 25th June 2011, we set off in Paul's van for Yate Park where the festival was being held (all the best bands turn up in a van). MLC had arrived! This was to be best yet. There was plenty of time before we were due to go on, so we made our way to the back stage area, where I met up with my sister and brother-in-law, who had come to support me.

We all had the jitters and needed to go to the loo, but we were running out of time as the act that was playing were nearly at the end of their set. Being a farmer's son, I took the brave decision to go behind a hedge to relieve the discomfort. That was where the diesel generator was and I quite expected to go up in a blue flash and a puff of smoke!

Then we saw the last act coming down the ladder from the stage, as this performance was to be from the back of a lorry. It was time to go on. We clambered up the vertical ladder and WE WERE

ON! No time to be nervous now.

The set we chose was:

1) Sticking Together: Brian Ferry

2) Dakota: Stereophonics

3) Road to Hell: Chris Rea

4) Have you Ever Fallen in Love: The Buzzcocks

5) No Matter What: Badfinger

6) Ziggy Stardust: David Bowie

7) Go Buddy Go: Stranglers

8) Whatever You Wanna Do: Eddie and the Hotrods

9) Back in the Night: Dr. Feelgood

10) China Girl: David Bowie.

Then, after five months of hard work putting it together, it was all over. We were told later on that the gate had been 3,000 that afternoon, something that I will never forget.

Having conquered Yate, MLC kept on going. We got our next gig the following October at the King William pub in Warmley, Bristol. This was to be our last, as Jacky's mother sadly died that December, and quite naturally she felt unable to carry on. Not long after that I heard that Jacky had got cancer. I did meet her once after that to hear that her treatment for it appeared to have been successful, but sadly the following summer the cancer returned, and she passed away. We had tried to recruit a keyboard player the previous year, but that plan fell through. Peter, Paul and I carried on playing, but only at open mic nights as when we had first met at the Portcullis in 2008.

My experience with the band taught me that despite my sensory limitations I was able to communicate with at least three other people who had no such restrictions on them. Now in 2014 and several pubs later, I still go to these open mic nights. The current one is at the Red Lion, Staple Hill in Bristol. This city is so fortunate to be blessed with so much musical talent. You can go out any night of the week and find live music being performed somewhere.

Meeting other people at the open mic sessions became a regular occurrence. The next person whose acquaintance I made was a professor in science and history in the shape of Alan Jocelyn. Alan was and still is a big Tom Petty fan, and I was recruited to be his drummer. The rudiments for these Petty songs were quite easy and fitted my learning curve, which was not too steep at the time.

CHAPTER 12

A new millennium

We were now at the turn of the century and a new millennium. Since I began writing this story of my life so many more things have happened, so there is more to be told.

Up until now I had come from living in the dark of the womb, then being born, still in a dark place, to being taken to hospital and given some sight, which made all the difference to my life.

In 1999, the press were in a whirl because there were stories going around that the world would collapse around their ears because of a computer virus linked to computer clocks which would get confused at the moment of switch-over to the year

2000 So far, I am still waiting for them to crash! Another bit of fake news. There was even a leaflet put through every letterbox explaining what was going to happen, and on the front was a picture of a computer chip with a menacing pair of eyes and crooked legs on it.

So that was how this century began. At that time I still had some sight left, though it had deteriorated somewhat and everything appeared like a fine mist. It did interfere with reading print, particularly if it was very small, like the smallest two sizes of newsprint. It did not stop me riding my motorbike out to places like Chipping Sodbury, or even into town, though that was a bit risky.

At home things were easier as I was out of direct sunlight, and for instance watching TV was not a problem. Cooking I had no difficulty with, but it was of a very basic nature – I lived by microwave!

At that time I was still at Snowdon Rd and was not considering a move, but then my younger sister Mary thought it might be better for me to move to Cardiff where they could help me now that my sight was failing. The move unfortunately did not work out, so I went back to Exeter. I tried going back to the farm, but that was a disaster as well.

By 2003 I was back in Fishponds, but I had made some friends at the Exeter Amateur Radio Club and we kept in touch by radio and phone, which has lasted to this day.

Comfort

One problem had still not gone away. There was still something missing in my life: a 'special relationship'. I had made a lot of acquaintances over the years, but that kind of friendship still eluded me. A visit to my GP resulted in a referral to a charitable organisation called Ways to Wellbeing. What really needed to be sorted out were my social skills, which up until then were abysmal or at least inadequate.

The man who came to my rescue was Stefano Mangoody, an Italian who was skilled in social management. We met up, and over coffee we talked about my problems and he said he would try to help with them. There was no group to begin with then but gradually, people began to join us at various coffee houses in Fishponds.

After about two years there were enough of us to fill up two tables, around 10 or 12 members. I was given a communicator guide whose job was to listen to the other members of the group and help me with contacting them. There were several others in that group whose problems were very different from mine. I could not make eye contact, so what with that and the hearing issues progress was slow at first. But after a year had passed I had learned what most people take for granted.

From that group of people I made three friends who are still around. One is Richard, who has a car, and we have done a few trips out and still meet in a local café. Another is Michael, who is very fond of his two dogs and is interested in films and musical stage performances, and another is Susanne, who I have not seen recently.

The Marmalade Trust

During my time at Ways to Wellbeing I was

introduced to one of the support workers, who told me about a charity called the Marmalade Trust. This charity enabled people who lived alone to go out on Christmas Day for a Christmas dinner. After a short phone call I was enrolled and on the 25th December a volunteer called and took me by car to the venue in a nearby pub. There were quite a lot of guests there ready for lunch. The menu was quite varied, catering for all kinds of dietary requirements, I went for the traditional menu, except for the fact that it needed to be suitable for a diabetic. The atmosphere was quite jolly and was rather like i imagined it to be in the Women's Institute! At the end of the lunch each of the guests was given a Christmas hamper. Whilst I did not make friends with anyone at the meal, it was nice to be invited.

Dave, the human guide dog

Being quite busy as I had become, I was in need of more mobility. Around 2016 I got in touch with the Guide Dogs Association about my needs, having tried the RNIB, who did not seem to have an option other than training me for a guide dog, which I did not think I would be able to deal with.

The Guide Dogs Association had a new scheme they were rolling out called the Ambassador Service. This service was quite new and they agreed to assess me for suitability. A member of their team came to see me and after going for a trial along the back lane behind the flats she said that she thought I would be suitable for being paired with a sighted guide who would be able to take me to various places around Bristol.

The plan was put into action and my volunteer guide was trained and CRB checked. The process took nearly 12 months to complete, but finally it was 'all systems go'. The day arrived and I was introduced to Dave. The team who had matched us had done their homework and the match was an extremely good one.

Dave had an interest in music, as do I. He liked church musical performances and some older rock genre styles and jazz. Although we have slightly different tastes, that did not seem to matter too much. He is still helping me.

Dave is my age, so he thinks on much the same lines as I do. We enjoy going to town and seeking out music stores and charity shops for bargain DVDs etc, and a few other places such as the City Farm at Windmill Hill, which until I met Dave I had never visited before.

Just over a year ago Dave took me to see a show at the Hippodrome called 'Motown', a musical about the life of Diana Ross. Dave's connections with the musical world are plenty, and he then introduced me to people at the Trinity Centre in Old Market Street. Once there I met some people who played reggae, led by a partially sighted guy called Barrington Chambers, who was in a full-time reggae band. With what I knew about drumming I was soon able to play some reggae and some ska. The Trinity Centre is a base for all the performing arts and I continued going there for 18 months, but because of the corona pandemic it sadly had to close in 2020. Looking back I did make it to the big stage – maybe one day it will be the pyramid.

Each trip ends with a lovely cup of tea, something

that Dave and I really enjoy, and best of all, this guide dog loves a natter!

Florida

Up until 1982, I had never flown across the pond to America. I had an acquaintance who I had met at Saint Loyes college, Exeter. who liked the idea, so we decided to go once our courses had ended. Savings were ring fenced, passports updated and bags packed. Another first was the Jumbo jet. Boeing 747s were well established aircraft, but neither of us had been on one.

The day arrived and we set off for the New World. Would it be as I had imagined? We were going to Florida as opposed to say New York, which everyone is familiar with, thanks to its skyscrapers. This was a holiday resort, sand and sea. The flight did seem rather long, a bit like what one of the Beatles described, 'turn left at Greenland.' It seemed to go on and on.

Finally we were stacking over Miami Airport, another first for me. On landing there was the novelty of seeing steam on the portholes due to the heat and the damp atmosphere. Our motel was right by the beach, so nothing could have been more convenient. What struck me about this place at Sun Isle was the cleanliness. The Americans definitely were very much aware of appearances, and still are, it seems.

We did one major side trip, to Cape Canaveral. The first shuttle was being launched in 10 days' time, and what a shame it was that we would have to miss such a spectacular event. The little shuttle bus took us all around the launch site, including an exhibition of moon rock, a lunar landing module and outside, some rockets, including a Mercury Redstone and a Saturn 5. We were also shown the VAB (vehicle assembly building), which was tall as a skyscraper, and the runway being prepared for the shuttle landings.

CHAPTER 13

Closing thoughts

Confidence

Now I have said quite a bit about confidence. It's something which was sadly missing in my youth but in the 21st century it returned as I became more mature. Someone I have been acquainted with for more than 40 years once said that I was 'a miserable old sod', but I beg to disagree with that person.

There is a charity called SENSE whose sole purpose is to help people who have been effected by the rubella virus to have a tolerable level of life. Talking with Sense put everything into perspective.

They told me that you learn about 80% of what you know through your eyes, which leaves 20 or thereabouts for the rest of your senses. They also told me that if sight was worth say a value of 10, and hearing was worth 10, then the total value of what you have lost would add up to 25, in other words more than the sum of the total. So when a person suffering with rubella mixes with a crowd of other people, unless they know and understand you, you are going to be a very lonely person feeling extremely isolated indeed.

The Department of Work and Pensions classified my sensory loss as 'severe'. I do experience a lot of frustration and prefer to be on my own to avoid the confrontations of conversation, i.e. people will ask me a question and many times I will have to say, 'can you repeat that please?' and if I don't hear it again, they will say 'oh never mind' and just walk away, no patience about the situation. I often wonder might have happened if my hearing had not been impaired. Maybe there could have been the beginning of a beautiful relationship.

Can you hear a smile?

I ask this question as there is a saying in the world of the blind that you cannot hear a smile. When you lose your sight, you gradually lose the aesthetics of life, like a lovely view, or say seeing an attractive person or garden etc. Bit by bit all the image information is being taken away like the layers of an onion. You are left with sounds of course, but if someone comes and sits down next to you and does not announce their presence to you, can you hear them smile?

My usual experience of this situation is when I have been sitting for a while and decide to leave, at which point the person who has been near will begin to speak just as I get up to put my coat on and leave!

There are many misunderstandings arising out of visual impairment. My favourite one is when I ask someone where something is, and they point and say, 'it's over there.' Sometimes when I am in the right frame of mind and feel a wind-up coming on I reply, 'where is over there?' Happily though, the majority of people are pretty helpful. The worst type is the yob. He or she can be verbally abusive and sometimes can physically obstruct you. People like this are usually in the 15 to 25-year-old category.

Funny folk

Not all comics are men. My all-time funny person is – or was until she sadly died – is Victoria Wood. Her humour was so down -to-earth, like her story about the Christmas stay over at a friend's house in the north of England. I can recommend it as it is 'traditional!' She did another one about supermarkets, and employed exaggeration as the tool to make you laugh.

Another funny person who I used to enjoy and who is also sadly no longer with us was Kenny Everett. Very dependent on visuals, rather like a comic strip at times, he always made me laugh, which I don't do all that often. To this list must be added Dame Edna (Barry Humphries). I don't like drag acts as a rule but this 'lady' gets me in stitches.

Films

There are not many films that I can really say I would watch more than once, but the Stanley Kubrick epic 2001, A Space Odyssey does take a lot of figuring out. Compression of time combined with all those weird colours, and the screaming sound track really does blow your mind the first time you watch it. The portrait of HAL the computer was so accurate. Now we have mobile phones that can comment on some of your questions, which is uncanny, and the prediction of flat TV displays too. One thing Kubrick could not portray properly was how the Earth would look from space, as there were no photographs of Earth from space at the time the film was made (1968), so it would have been better to have left that shot out.

The trilogy 'Back to the Future' is another bit of sci-fi in my collection – it's a pity I can't see it any more. Classic films should include 'Gandhi'. I think it was Barry Norman, the TV film critic, who told how when the script was being looked at said one producer read it and said 'who wants to make a movie about a man dressed in a bed sheet who carries a bean pole around with him?' This producer obviously did not have a sense of history.

The end game

Trying to summarise one's life when hopefully there is more to come can be a difficult task. At the time of completing this book I am just approaching my 73rd birthday. It would be very easy to say that it has been a hard, frustrating life, as we all experience disappointment and frustration from time to time. My early life was good compared to those of some people. For instance I was born to hard-working, intelligent parents who were faced with a child who had been badly affected by the rubella virus. There were times during my teens when so much uncertainty surrounded me that things could have been far worse. For example, victims of rubella have a mortality rate of 20% during their teenage years. I was lucky to survive and go on to see adulthood.

In my 20s and 30s I saw most of my friends get

married. At that time I felt very lonely and isolated, but now I am older and I hope wiser, I have come to appreciate that maybe married life would not have been the best thing for me.

Trust

Often during conversations about faith and trust, words which we use in regard to our feelings about religion, we put a lot of emphasis on 'trust.' How can I trust God when I know of so many people who have suffered? It must take a lot of faith to overcome some of the wrong doings by the powers-that-be.

God to most people is some invisible entity, and they say something is just 'God's will' to get around the issue of something that quite clearly is wrong. As far as I am concerned, God has too many escape clauses and caveats in his contract with us. My definition of God is just a combination of chemistry, biology and physics with a dash of randomness thrown in it. If I sound a bit negative in my attitude, well I am, and I doubt if that will change very much.

The world starts to fade

When you are told by an eye consultant that you are losing your sight it fills you with apprehension. In 1989 the head man at Bristol eye infirmary tried me with contact lenses to try and make the most of the sight that I had. The results of the test were very encouraging. I could see down to the red line, which is the bench mark for 20/20 vision. Unfortunately the lenses would not stay in place because my eyes are not spherical, so that was that. I was given some drops to reduce the effects of glaucoma, but the inevitable was going to happen one day. By 2000 the effects were beginning to show, and my life was changing.

Of course I sometimes imagine what my children would have been like. Of course, I wonder how they would have progressed during their lives, but they may have got into bad company, which would have caused me and my partner a lot of anxiety. I have never been without a roof over my head. Many of our young people today are not so fortunate as they have very little chance of owning a home of their own, but live in the rented sector on short tenancy contracts, which must make them feel very insecure.

Employment has been a difficult aspect of my life. There were very few kinds of employment that I was considered suitable for me. The farm was an option, but small was no longer beautiful in the late 1960s and early 1970s. It was a case of 'get big or get out.' My hope of doing electronics was dashed of course when I went to the tv manufacturer in Plymouth where it was discovered that I could not see the value rings on a 1/4 watt resistor. These components were only as thick as the wires at either end of them, making it difficult for people with 20 20 vision to see them, never mind me!

Conversely, I had to learn to live on a low budget, as a result I have survived some of the problems which I could have had when paying for expensive replacement items such as washing machines etc.

My life now seems to be 'set fair,' I have lived in this flat now for nine years, I have got a circle of very good friends and still have my three sisters. The music goes on as usual, and there is still some hope that I shall get another band to drum for, despite my age.

BV - #0082 - 030821 - C4 - 203/127/9 - PB - 9781861519801 - Gloss Lamination